Is it Mold?

A Holistic Approach to Managing a Commonly Overlooked Condition

Karen Wright, MS

DISCLAIMER: The medical statements or information provided in this literature are for educational purposes only. It is recommended that this information be used in conjunction with a visit to a qualified health care professional.

No action should be taken by the reader based solely on the contents of this book. The natural treatments and suggestions discussed here can affect different people in different ways. Occasionally adverse reactions might occur. Readers who fail to consult appropriate health authorities assume the risk of any injuries.

Since there are constant changes resulting from ongoing research and clinical experience, some of the literature presented may not be current. The author and the publisher are not responsible for errors and/or omissions.

The purpose of this book is to provide information that will educate the reader to make more informed health and dietary choices.

DEDICATION

To my daughter Mara and my son Alex who never stop believing in me and support me through all the ups and downs that I have experienced in the process of writing this book, including when my computer crashed and I lost everything and had to start writing the book from scratch.

CONTENTS

ACKNOWLEDGMENTS

This book is part of my own thirteen year journey to solve health issues caused by toxic exposure after the September 11, 2001 attacks on the World Trade Center. My own road to recovery was not an easy one. There were many roadblocks that caused my health to turn for the worse. I spent much of the time during my illness reading, studying and trying many new options that only partially worked but I kept persevering until I started feeling better. I gained so much knowledge that I decided to leave my corporate America computer programming job and return to school to obtain the credentials needed to help other people with their own health journeys. I learned more in school as I earned a traditional Doctor of Naturopathy degree and a Masters in Human Nutrition and Functional Medicine.

It is while getting my Masters that I learned about Mold Sensitivity Syndrome. One of my classes was neuroendocrinology taught by Dr. David H. Haase. For the class we had to write a paper from a list of different topics. There were none that really interested me so I randomly selected Mold Sensitivity Syndrome. The more I researched the more I became fascinated about this condition and related to people who have it. After becoming toxic from the September 11th debris, entering any building or area that had a mold condition would send my health spiraling in a downward motion. I read study after study about the trials and tribulations of people with this condition. I combed PubMed to find solutions to the problem. I tested protocols on myself and became a building mold detective. If it had not been for Dr. David H. Haase this book would never have been written. It was his inspiration that encouraged me to explore the complexity of health conditions and look for solutions that are not considered a standard part of conventional medicine.

Just looking at the journey I have travelled to accomplish the success with my own health has taught me that there are numerous possibilities, some will work for some people and others will not. I also learned never to give up hope. It was through my hope and the support of my friends and family that I was able to restore my own health.

Though I have never had direct contact with Dr. Ritchie Shoemaker, his research laid the foundation for helping and identifying people with mold disease. His clinical expertise has helped many people with this condition. Dr. Shoemaker was the starting point for my research on this condition.

I thank Dr. Walter Crinnion for teaching me about detoxification and giving me the understanding of the biological processes involved in detoxifying one's body.

Dr. Alex Vasquez is an amazing teacher and practitioner. Using his five part protocol I was able to refine my process for restoring my health when exposed to mold. Though I could never keep up with him in the amount of scientific research I read, he taught me the importance of good scientific research and how to tell the difference between good and bad research.

Laura Keiles, one of my colleagues and a fellow author helped by reviewing the validity and giving suggestions from her area of expertise. Her book "Foodergies" is a reference book to help people overcome food sensitivities and/or allergies and may be of interest to readers of this book. She was inspirational in bringing this project to completion.

I would like to thank the person from www.auroradesigner.com who designed the cover.

Wendy Stout generously shared her photos of her home mold remediation project.

This book could not have been completed without the help of my friends and other members of my family. Immense thanks to Robin Wright, Alexander and Mara Felman, Erica Wright and Bohdan Mykulak who each spent countless hours proof reading and making suggestions to help improve the content of the book and cooking nutritious meals while I worked diligently to get the book completed.

Terri Leinneweber has been a true friend since I met her while working in corporate America. She spent hours proofing the book and questioning anything that did not make sense. Without her time and dedication I am not sure this book would have been completed.

My friends from Institute of Integrative Nutrition and Spotlight kept me motivated to complete this book. Special thanks to Lindsey Smith, Joshua Rosenthal, Shannon Vogel and Blue Russ for the encouragement and help.

After September 11 my goal was to get healthy and remove my pain. I did this through diet and lifestyle changes. Though September 11 was an unusual toxic load I was able to repeatedly stabilize my health after every setback. It is my honor to share my efforts with you.

To your abundant health –

Karen Wright
Traditional Naturopath, Functional Nutritionist and Health Coach
December 2014

1 INTRODUCTION

Recently there has been a lot of media attention concerning removing gluten from the diet. Gluten is found in many grain products including but not limited to wheat, rye, and barley. You probably know at least one person that has been told to avoid gluten. The supermarket shelves are well stocked with many new products that are gluten-free. For people with wheat sensitivities avoiding wheat might be challenging until the person figures out all the hidden sources of gluten. Gluten can be found in odd places like some lipsticks or the seal used on many commercial tea bags. These accidental exposures can cause a person who can't have gluten to experience health issues. In most instances the person can learn what to avoid and can have control over the condition.

But, imagine that you were sensitive to something that was not easy to avoid and like gluten if you did not avoid it, your health would negatively spiral downward leaving you unable to function. People with mold sensitivity syndrome are in this position, as avoiding mold is not an easy task. Each time a person enters a building there is a possibilty that mold lurking in it will cause their health to tailspin. Unlike products containing gluten, there is no label on any building saying mold-free.

A person seeking medical help, will find that the medical community is not designed to look for the cause of the illness but to patch the symptoms. People are often told by medical practitioners that mold can't make you sick. If the practitioner had just looked at the pattern of the condition, they may have realized that mold illness is a true condition. Slight exposure to mold can make many people feel a little ill but for some people it can be a crippling experience. Mold sensitivity is often misdiagnosed as various other conditions because of the belief that mold cannot cause disease.

However, mold sensitivity syndrome is a real condition and if the true cause of the disease is not identified, the person will get sicker and sicker each time they walk into a mold infested building. Unfortunately, for people with mold sensitivity each exposure makes the condition worse and triggers an autoimmune response.

Avoidance is not always feasible; there are some measures to control the home environment that can help people with this condition. As a result of implementing these measures, when entering a building which contains mold, they are not as severely knocked off their feet. It is important to have a safe home to return to for healing.

For people who have been sick and cannot find the cause, mold may the culprit. For example, I had a client who got sick every time it rained. She was told that was due to recurring Lyme disease. To me it seemed strange that the Lyme kept recurring after a heavy rainfall. I asked my client if she could think of any place where there might be exposure to mold. It turned out that the basement in her house was getting flooded whenever it rained, which caused a mold condition. Fixing the water leak and accurately cleaning the mold helped the client immensely and her "Lyme" went away. This is only one client. For another person it may not be the mold that is causing the problem but actually Lyme causing the disease. The point is to look for a pattern that occurs with any condition. By looking at the problem differently another solution may appear.

This book is meant to be used to help people struggling with a condition that could be caused by mold. After the September 11 attacks to the World Trade Center, I became extremely ill from the toxic exposure. Since that time I have struggled with sensitivities to many things, mold being one of them. I have had to implement the techniques described in this book to help myself. Unfortunately, mold exposure can occur at anytime. The last time I had a mold attack was at the Portland, Oregon Airport. When I got off the plane I immediately got ill from the mold which had a very strong smell. I felt like the air was knocked out of me and started wheezing, my eyes watered and I felt awful in a matter of a few seconds. Going outside did not help as the mold was still present in the air. I had come a long way to a conference and needed to be able to function. This book will contain some of the things I have learned through coping with the condition, and the research of other practitioners who are treating people who have mold sensitivity. The design of the book is to help you ask the right questions and help the treating physician find new ways to help you regain your health.

2 DESCRIPTION AND HISTORY OF CONDITION

"Mold" is defined in Merriam Webster's dictionary as a superficial, often woolly growth, produced especially on damp or decaying organic matter or on living organisms by a fungus (as of the order Mucorales). ("Definition of MOLD," 2013). Mold is a type of fungus. In this book, I will often use mold to reference the above definition. There are a few instances, however, when it will be referred as fungus; this because of the nature of the research used in that part of the text. Mold is something that most people have come in contact with at some point during their lifetime. The most common occurrence for many people is forgotten wet laundry in the washing machine. Hopefully this doesn't occur on a hot day when the awful smell is stronger. In that instance opening the washing machine does not bring the usual smell of clean clothes but an awful one and that smell is mold. Although this is an annoying experience it does not cause a problem for everybody. However, for people with Mold Sensitivity Syndrome, any exposure to mold can set off a cascade of events.

Mold Sensitivity Syndrome is a serious illness caused by an immune response to decaying organic matter. Mold sensitivity is not an allergy. It causes a different kind of immunological response than an allergy. However, forgotten wet laundry in the washer is not the usual type of exposure that causes mold illness. Most often the illness is triggered by a mold condition that is inside a building usually caused by damage from a leak, but it can be triggered by outside mold as well. Unlike the wet laundry, the mold conditions are often not easy to identify.

When mold is inhaled through the nose, a person with mold illness reacts with acute and chronic inflammatory response to multiple biotoxins that have taken up residence inside a water damaged building.

Sick Building Syndrome (SBS) is another name often associated with mold sensitivity syndrome. But Sick Building Syndrome can also be caused by plasticizers, formaldehyde and microbial volatile organic compounds

(MVOC). Volatile organic compounds (VOC) are chemicals that have a low molecular weight, low water solubility and high vapor pressure. Because of these characteristics VOC can easily evaporate into the air. When a microbe produces a VOC it is called a MVOC. Research has shown the MVOC's are higher in homes with reported dampness and mold. (Sahlberg et al., 2013)

For the purposes of this book, a sick building is any structure where water damage has resulted in mold growth. Water and cellulose are the two main ingredients needed for mold to grow. Cellulose is found in dust particles. Water can come from a variety of sources. The obvious ones are leaky pipes, rainwater and condensation on pipes. In the right environment, mold will grow. Fungus divides rapidly, reproducing itself once every thirty minutes. With the right conditions, at that rate, it will not take long before a building has a widespread mold problem. (Shoemaker, 2010)

Mold plays an important role in the outside environment by helping to breakdown dead organic matter like leaves. To reproduce, mold creates many tiny spores. Some of the spores can float in the air. When the spores land on a wet surface they begin to grow. Many types of mold have been identified. All of them require water or moisture to grow. The spores cannot be seen until they form large colonies. Because mold is not visible until the colonies have formed, smell is often the first sense used to identify mold. Food is a good example of a mold colony formation. On moldy bread or fruit the visible portion of the mold are the colonies that have formed.

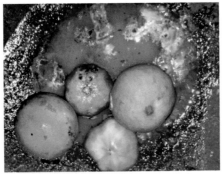

Food Mold Colony

Historically, mold is not a new problem. As a matter of fact, the problem of mold in buildings can be traced back to the Old Testament of the Bible where it was referred to as "plague". The Book of Leviticus 14:

33-53, described specific instructions for finding, removing and remediating mold. The process of determining existence of mold was described in Leviticus 14:33-39:

> *And the LORD spoke unto Moses and unto Aaron, saying,*
> *When ye be come into the land of Canaan, which I give to you*
> *for a possession, and I put the plague of leprosy in a house of the land*
> *of your possession; And he that owneth the house shall come and tell*
> *the priest, saying, It seemth to me there is as it were a plague in the*
> *house: Then the priest shall command that they empty the house,*
> *before the priest go into it to see the plague, that all that is in the*
> *house be not made unclean: and afterward the priest shall go in to see*
> *the house: And he shall look on the plague, and behold, if the plague*
> *be in the walls of the house with hollow streaks, greenish or reddish,*
> *which in sight are lower than the wall; Then the priest shall go out of*
> *the house to the door of the house and shut up the house seven days:*
> *And the priest shall come again the seventh day, and shall look:*
> *and, behold, if the plague be spread in the walls of the house;*

Though there is no way to tell what type of mold was being described in Leviticus, the mold in the passage has greenish or red color. Coincidently, Stachybotrys, one of the most common molds found in homes today, is a greenish-black color.

The next passages Leviticus 14: 39-42 describe the instructions for plague removal after the seven day quarantine has ended which includes complete removal of the infected stones and replacement with new ones. The infected stones are to be discarded in an area that is remote from city; this will preserve the sanitary conditions of the area.

> *The priest shall command that they take away the stones in*
> *which the plague is, and they shall cast them into an unclean place*
> *without the city: And he shall cause the house to be scraped within*
> *round about, and they shall pour out the dust that they scrape off*
> *without the city into an unclean place: And they shall take other*
> *stones, and put them in the place of those stones; and he shall take*
> *other mortar, and shall plaster the house.*

If the mold condition returned after all the precautions were taken, the house is then destroyed and the debris is put in an area that is remote from the city. The persons who lived in the house would have to thoroughly clean themselves and the clothes that they wore while in the house. This process is described in Leviticus 14: 43-47

> *And if the plague come again, and break out in the house, after that he hath taken away the stones, and after he hath scraped the house, and after it is plastered. Then the priest shall come and look, and, behold, if the plague be spread in the house, it is a fretting leprosy in the house: it is unclean. And he shall break down the house, the stones of it, and the timber thereof, and all the mortar of the house; and he shall carry them forth out of the city into an unclean place. Moreover, he that goeth into the house all the while that it is shut up shall be unclean until the even. And he that lieth in the house shall wash all his clothes; and he that eateth in the house shall wash his clothes.*

Finally, there are instructions for a cleaning ritual if it has been determined that the mold had no longer spread throughout the house. Cedar wood, hyssop, scarlet and two birds were used to accomplish the cleaning. Cedar oil is a natural product that has been used for mold and mildew elimination. The oil naturally kills fungus, microbes and spores. It is effective for removing mold from stone and preventing new mold growth. The hyssop referenced in the bible is thought to be origanum syriacum which is a member of the mint family. It has antibacterial, antifungal and antispasmodic properties. (Bakkour et al, 2011) The cedar and the hyssop could be used as an essential oil blend. Scarlet referred to red dyed wool, which during Biblical times, was considered to have antimicrobial properties. The combination of all the ingredients could be used to make an antibacterial soap. The passage for the cleansing is from Leviticus 14:48-53

> *And if the priest shall come in, and look upon it, and, behold, the plague hath not spread in the house, after the house is plastered; then the priest shall pronounce the house clean, because the plague is healed. And he shall take to cleanse the house two birds, and cedar wood, and scarlet, and hyssop: And he shall kill the one of the birds*

in an earthen vessel over running water: And he shall take the cedar wood, and the hyssop, and the scarlet and the living bird and dip them in the blood of the slain bird, and in the running water and sprinkle the house seven times: And he shall cleanse the house with the blood of the bird, and with the running water and with the living bird and with the cedar wood and with the hyssop and with the scarlet: But he shall let go of the living bird out of the city into the open fields, and make atonement for the house: and it shall be clean.

The specific instructions to remediate mold do not vary much from the current recommended protocol. There was a concern about keeping people far away from the mold and disposing the contaminated building material in a manner that it did not affect people living in the city. This concern indicates that people during that time period were getting ill from mold.

3 THE NEW FACE OF MOLD

Since mold and its disease have been a problem for a really long time, why are more and more people suddenly becoming seriously ill with this disease? Since biblical times, new products have been introduced to prevent fungus and building construction has changed. Though many modern day inventions may be useful tools, they have created a mold problem that is greater than that seen in biblical times. In recent years there have been many storms that have caused flooding and damage to buildings. Oftentimes after these storms, people are anxious to return to their homes and/or have limited funds, leading them to cut corners in removing the mold and the mold condition remains.

The mold epidemic started around the 1970s and has been escalating at a rapid pace ever since. Interestingly, the term Sick Building Syndrome was not coined until the mid-1970s. One of the products introduced in 1970 was an antifungal product, Benlate, made by DuPont for use by farmers. The active component of Benlate is benomyl. Benlate was the most successful fungicide ever made by DuPont. In the first year, many farmers were happy with the product. For farmers, fungus is a big problem since it can quickly destroy crops. The success of Benlate meant greater crop yield for the farmer which resulted in greater profits. In the years that followed the farmers' experience was different. The second year, the farmers had less success and every year after the benefit diminished until eventually farmers lost their entire crops and could no longer use their land. Losing an entire farm because of this chemical fungicide angered the farmers and they sued DuPont. After many law suits DuPont stopped making Benlate, though the company still claims the product is safe. The reason for the crop destruction is that each year some of the fungi survived spraying. The fungus that survived mutated and became resistant to Benlate. Since fungal organisms reproduce quickly, adaptation is much easier and quicker than in organisms like humans that don't reproduce often. Because Benomyl disrupts the normal transfer of chromosomes when cells divide, not only did the fungi mutate but the mutation led to behavioral change as well. The new fungi had no competition from other organisms and rapidly took over new territory. These new fungal organisms are resistant to fungicides. The DNA of a new fungus has the ability to transfer to cell dividing organisms. (Shoemaker, 2010, p. 274) This feature makes these fungi extremely dangerous since it can spread from living creature to living creature. Fungi called Fusarium oxysporum schlecht and the Pseudomonas flourescens bacteria were found in the areas that had been sprayed. In places that had not been treated these are rarely found. Cyanide was released by the microbes that were sprayed with Benlate and ended up killing plants in the area through the roots. Pseudomonas flourescens is resistant to cyanide but the plants are not. The fungi, bacteria, and cyanide pose a huge health risk to people living close to sprayed areas. The fact that DuPont stopped producing Benlate does not change the mutated fungi. They will go on reproducing for many years. Based on the research of Dr. Ritchie Shoemaker, who is recognized as a leader in the field of biotoxin related illness, the mutated fungi also produce toxins. (http://www2.dupont.com/Phoenix_Heritage/en_US/1970_detail.html; Shoemaker, 2010)

At the same time that Benlate was introduced, another new product hit the market: Lucite Paints, which also contains benomyl to prevent fungal growth in the home. This paint was supposed to control Aureobasidium pullulans. Any home painted with the fungal paint that gets water damage would end up with the mutated fungus. Benomyl is still being added to paint. The following mutated benomyl resistant fungi can be found inside water damaged buildings: Fusarium, Trichoderma, Aspergillus nidulans, Aspergillus parasiticus, Penicillium citrinum, Penicillium chrysogenum, Acremonium chrysogenum, Aspergillus flavus, Penicillium italicum and Penicillium digitatum. (Shoemaker, 2009; Shoemaker, 2010) Many people paint bathrooms or basements with antifungal paint. Since many of these paints contain benomyl, it is possible for mutated fungus to grow in those locations. Since the mutated fungus have a changed behavior from non mutated fungus they are difficult to remove. Unfortunately, many consumers are not aware that this can pose a problem. For someone who has Sick Building Syndrome this is an even bigger issue. Imagine thinking that you are preventing the mold which makes you sick by using mold preventing paint and in actuality, the paint will produce mutated mold that will make you sicker and be hard to remediate. For a person with mold sensitivity any exposure to mold is a problem. I personally would not use antifungal paint. Even if the antifungal paint does not contain benomyl, until there is scientific evidence that no antifungal agent used causes fungal mutations, I would rather play it safe than be sorry later. Acrylic paints are better to use than oil paints. Some species of molds can survive on the ingredients of oil paints.

Modern building construction adds another dimension to the problem. In 1970 there was an oil crisis. In order to save energy, new buildings were designed to reduce the amount of exchange between inside and outside air. This new design cut energy costs. New office buildings are being built with heating, ventilation and air conditioning (HVAC) systems for cooling and heating. HVAC systems were also being retrofitted into old buildings. If the wrong size unit is installed, installed improperly, or not properly maintained, problems will arise. Not only does the filter need to be changed regularly, but the right filter must to be used. For people with mold sensitivity the highest level minimum efficiency reporting value (MERV) filter should be used, which currently is sixteen. As more electronic equipment has been introduced into the work place, the HVAC unit needs to address the extra demand caused by the additional heat from the electronics. It is better to overestimate the HVAC needed than to purchase one that is too small. Having a HVAC that can handle the additional electrical load as new gadgets come onto the market will allow for the HVAC to be more effective in the future. Many people have installed HVAC units in their homes. As more electronics are added to the home the size of the unit may not be correct.

If there is a major leak in the building the air needs to flow well to prevent mold formation. In many office buildings the windows cannot be opened. Without being able to open the windows when there is a leak, the building will not get aired out suitably and mold is more likely to form. In homes that have HVAC units, windows are opened less frequently.

HVAC units are problems for both commercial and residential buildings with ventilation issues, if the wrong type of unit is installed. Regular maintenance to replace the filter with a proper one must occur for these units to keep the air clean. If you have a unit in the home that was installed a few years ago, have a professional check to see if the unit still fulfills the needs of your home with the current electric load and if it can handle any additional load for future technology advances.

Window air conditioners collect dust and moisture on the air ducts, drain pan, and coils. This combination is a formula for mold. Running the air conditioners about 10 minutes on humid days can help prevent mold from occurring. Also, vacuuming the window air conditioner with a high-efficiency particulate absorption (HEPA) filter vacuum can clean the dust and help prevent the mold environment. The front plate on the units is removable to make it possible to clean. Make sure not to miss the drain pan during the cleaning process.

Windows can also cause problems. Broken seals allow condensation to get into the home. Check for broken seals and replace them as needed.

Heavy rain or snow can cause a flat roof to bow, creating weak spots that allow water to seep into the building. If it is a slow leak it could be a long time before it is discovered. Since water travels easily, finding the leak can take awhile. Noticeable signs of the leak may not occur anywhere near the actual location of the leak. If there are dropped ceilings in the building it may take even longer before the leak is discovered due to the gap. The space between the actual ceiling and the dropped ceiling provides a breeding ground for mold. Unkempt or damaged roof gutters can result in a roof that leaks.

French drains are an exterior house addition, used to move surface water away from a building. These drains work well if they are well maintained. When not maintained they can be a source of mold contamination in the home. If the ground area closest to the house is slightly slanted away from the house this will prevent water from collecting around the foundation or entering into the home.

Paper insulation and dry wall material pose additional problems. Libraries have a similar problem with books that become moldy. When the dry wall material gets wet the wet section should be removed and replaced.

My dad was a structural engineer and was always complaining about the quality of modern homes not being built as sturdy as the old stock. There are probably many old buildings that also have construction flaws. I personally have multiple friends with custom built homes that were leaking from the day they took possession. Finding the location of the construction flaw can be like finding a needle in a haystack. There are other people that I know with sump pumps in their basement to remove water after a rain storm. The pumps only work if there is electricity. With storms like Hurricane Sandy knocking out power for days, one can only imagine what is growing inside those homes. If you have mold sensitivity, buying a home that requires a sump pump is not a good idea.

Another modern day addition to both offices and homes is wall to wall carpet. If something spills on the carpet it is impossible to completely dry it. The carpet now becomes a perfect mold breeding ground. Besides the possibility of the carpet becoming moldy, carpets in general are not good for anyone that has allergies. Carpets collect of a lot of microscopic dust and debris. Vacuuming doesn't remove all of the debris. A trick used by door to door vacuum cleaner sales people is to use a white handkerchief over the nozzle to show you how much dirt is on the carpet. They usually won't do it more than a second time in the same spot because they know it is impossible to get all the dirt up. The same problem can occur on couches and mattresses. Since the windows remain closed in homes with an HVAC system there is no way to air out the home as is needed.

Some modern day appliances, though convenient, are breeding grounds for mold. Front load washing machines add additional counter space but water often accumulates in the door gasket and rapidly breeds mold. As a mold prevention measure, leave the door open and remove the pooled water from the gasket seam. With busy schedules there is a possibilty of forgetting to leave the door open after switching the clothes to the dryer or not having time to remove the pooled water and the washer now breeds mold. Running a cycle with a quart of white vinegar and hot water, no clothes, will clean the washing machine and might reduce the likelihood that mold forms in the gasket.

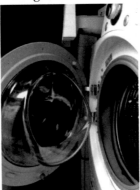

Front Load Washer Properly Aired After Use

The laundry room contains lots of lint and dust, adding water to the mixture makes this is a perfect place for mold to accumulate. Therefore if you have mold sensitivity and are thinking of buying a new washer do not get a front loader. If you have a front loading washing machine consider replacing it with a top loading machine. As mentioned earlier there is always the issue of forgetting clothes in the washer which than can become moldy.

If the dryer is not vented outside, the humidity created during the drying cycle can cause mold to form. This can be a problem for people living in apartments that use inside venting systems. These usually consist of a container that is filled with water at the end of the venting pipe. The container fills with the lint and the water prevents it from being flammable and getting all over the house. Some people have also used this technique so that the dryer becomes a source of heat. In reality what is happening is a lot of moist air is being added into the home in an area where there is a lot of dust and this becomes the prefect breeding ground for mold. Since there is water in the bucket to contain the lint, more moisture is being put inside the house and this creates an even bigger mold breeding ground. If you are not venting the dryer inside the home, the outside vent can still cause an issue. Venting pipes that travel a long distance before leaving the house can cause damp lint to deposit in the pipe. There are special fans that are specifically designed for dryer ducts that can help push the lint out and keep the pipe clear. A fan not designed specifically for use in dryer ducts will easily become ruined from the drying moisture and lint. A basement crawl space is not a good location for venting a dryer. This would cause moisture under the house which would result in mold.

Dryer vents may need insulation depending on where they are installed. If the vent is in an unheated basement or any place that gets cold, insulating the vent will prevent the moisture from freezing in the pipe. If the pipe gets frozen as the water thaws, it could lead to condensation on the pipe which in turn can create mold.

Underneath the refrigerator there are drip pans which are mold breeding grounds. Some refrigerators come with removable trays that can be cleaned, but many people don't know they exist. Moisture from the refrigerator condensation and food spills that go undetected can cause a mold condition. When cleaning the refrigerator, clean underneath it to prevent mold from accumulating.

The dish drying rack used for hand-washed dishes is another place where water can accumulate. After cleaning the dishes wipe the area down to prevent any possible growth. If you have a dish washer, as with the front loading washer, if there is any dampness after cleaning the dishes, leave the door ajar to prevent any mold growth.

In the winter the air is dry and some people use humidifiers to keep the air moist or even help with colds. Since there is plastic and steam in an enclosed container it is the perfect place for mold to grow. When I was a child, my parents used to put pots of water on the radiator to add moisture back into the air. The heat from the radiator evaporated the water. If you have the type of radiators that would allow a pot of water on top, that is preferable to the humidifier. Since the pot is not enclosed it is less likely to get moldy and it is easier to clean than a humidifier. Just clean the pot and put in fresh water on a daily basis to add moisture to the home.

Fireplaces smell wonderful and in some cases are the method used to heat the home. But if the chimney space is not maintained it will allow water to seep into the home and mold can grow. If you have a chimney check the flashing, bricks, and chimney caps for damage and fix as necessary. This can help prevent water from getting into the home. Sweeping the chimney helps to remove the mold and keep it free from creosote. Creosote is a gummy, combustible byproduct of wood burning that is formed when the volatile gases from the burning process combine and condense on the way out of the chimney. When the fireplace cools the gases solidify and the creosote is formed. Creosote causes most chimney fires. The chimney also works more efficiently when it is cleaned.

The basement is usually the source of many mold issues. The pipes in the basement, if not properly insulated, will have condensation on them during humid months. The basement can also be the place of flooding after heavy rainfalls or leaky pipes. Having a dehumidifier in the basement can help remove the extra water in the area. The best way to do this is to have someone run a pipe from the dehumidifier to the outside of the house so the water is easily eliminated from the house. The dehumidifiers that have to be emptied can create a problem if they are not emptied often enough.

Using materials like drywall instead of wood gives the mold a breeding ground. Drywall is much easier for mold to feed on than wood. The only way to remediate contaminated drywall is to cut out the infected piece and replace it. This is the exact removal process as described in the

Bible. If there is no obvious mold on the drywall but there are spots that have swelling or the seams of the walls are no longer intact, those areas should be replaced with new materials. Even if there is no mold in the swollen areas these are areas that could potentially have an issue.

Wallpaper is another modern invention that can potentially cause a mold condition if it gets wet. Since removing the section of wallpaper that is damaged is not always practical due to aesthetics, I suggest not using wallpaper especially for large areas.

The bathroom is an area that tends to get moldy. Having an exhaust fan or opening windows while taking a hot steaming shower will keep the area dryer. After the shower, spreading the shower curtain for drying will help prevent mold from forming in the curtains folds. Leave the windows and/or exhaust fan running until the bathroom is dry.

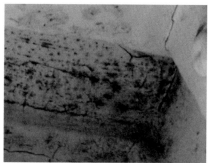

Black Mold on Ceiling of Improperly Vented Bathroom

4 REMEDIATING THE PROBLEM

1. Dry the area

If there has been any water damage from flooding or a leak the best course of action is to dry the area as soon as possible. In most cases mold will not form if the area is thoroughly dried within the first 24-48 hours. Dehumidifiers, fans, heaters and wet vacuums can be used. Wet vacuums can remove the bulk of the water. Air flow into the building is important. Open as many windows and doors as possible to circulate the air and dry any moisture.

Books, important documents, and papers may have to be thrown away. There are restoration specialists who might be able to save some of the documents. You can try drying books by putting something like a chop stick between every page to allow air to get between the pages and preventing them from sticking together as the book dries. A fan can be placed near the book so the pages dry quicker. Once the book is completely dried a heavy object may be needed to flatten the book.

Any curtains that were damaged should be cleaned based on the manufacturer's instructions. Cleaning upholstered furniture may pose a problem and require reupholstering if the frame is worth keeping. Any damaged or swollen dry wall needs to be completely replaced.

Moldy items should not be touched with bare hands and a face mask should be used to prevent breathing any possible spores.

2. Assess the mold damage

After the cleaning is in motion, assess the situation. Some questions to consider:
- Is there an existing moisture problem in the building?
- Are the materials still wet after more than 48 hours?
- Are there strong smelling moldy odors in the building?
- Where are the possible hidden sources of water?
- Is anyone experiencing any health issues? Are there new health issues? Have old issues unexplainably gotten worse?
- Is there visible damage to the building materials?

3. Create a plan

The plan should be very detailed so there is a clear set of instructions and no steps are missed. Being thorough prevents problems occurring after the remediation has been completed. Things to include in the remediation plan:

- Future mold prevention strategy
- Prevention of contamination to the rest of home
- Course of action if someone gets ill
- Expected timeframe and cost.

4. Implement the plan

With a clear plan, the implementation phase should run smoothly and the home will be free of mold again.

Problem

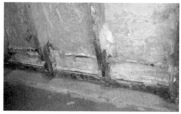

Mold Lower Part of Wall

Remediation

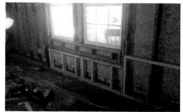

Complete Wall Board Removal

5 TESTING AND CLEANING MOLD

The Environmental Relative Moldiness Index (ERMI) is the test that was developed by the Environmental Protection Agency (EPA) as a tool to determine the potential health risks of indoor mold. To do the test, dust samples are collected from the building often using places that are known to have a mold problem, like a carpet. The test looks for a combination of thirty-six molds from two groups. The group that we are concerned with is the group that appears in buildings that have had water damage. The other group contains mold that is not caused by water damage. The results are based on a DNA analysis called Mold Specific Quantitative PCR (MSQPCR) which detects the presence of specific unique DNA sequences that have been found to be prevalent in mold damaged buildings. The building is given a number that is usually between negative ten and positive twenty and from that number it is grouped into one of four levels. The least amount of mold burden is an ERMI level of one. Four is the highest level which indicates the likelihood of mold in the building. According to Dr. Ritchie Shoemaker, for anyone that is susceptible to mold, the ERMI should be less than two. This test is a tool to evaluate the potential risk of indoor mold growth.

Environmental medicine expert, Dr. Walter Crinnion recommends that both the indoor and neighboring outdoor areas be tested for mold when samples are collected, since mold lives both indoors and outdoors. If the concentration of mold inside the home is greater than that outside of the home there is a mold problem that needs to be remediated. After the mold condition is remedied, the home should again be tested for mold. The retest should include not just the area that was remediated but adjoining areas as well. If the clean-up is not done correctly, there is a possibilty for cross contamination.

A qualified mold company would set up a machine in several places both inside and outside of the home. The machine collects the mold spores by moving air across a filter. After the sample has been collected, the particles that stick to the filter would be checked microscopically and counted. Other collection methods include using sticky tape to collect mold; removing part of the contaminated area and sending it to a lab and using Q-tips in different areas to collect the samples.

The company that tests for the mold and the company that cleans the mold should not be the same company. The person doing the testing should have no financial interest in or business relationship with the clean-up company. When the two companies have a vested interest in each other the result is likely to be more cost to the consumer for things that are not necessarily needed. Remediating mold can be costly but some of the cost should not be spent on things that are not an issue.

There are test kits that can be bought in the store but these only test the indoor levels and they cannot test all the molds. Stachybotrys, also called black mold, is one of the mold types that the kits do not pick up. Stachybotrys is a common mold that is often found in poorly vented bathrooms and laundry rooms.

An infrared inspection is a quick way to determine if there are any locations that have moisture where mold might be able to develop. Once detected, a moisture measuring meter can be used to determine the areas' moisture level. Any high reading is a good indication that there is mold growing in the area.

Since mold has a strong odor, dogs have been trained to find mold. Trained dogs can be useful in areas that are not accessible to people.

The American Industrial Hygiene Association (AIHA) and the American Conference of Governmental Industrial Hygienists (ACGIH) have recommendations about mold sampling protocols. Occasionally ACGIH offers workshops on Mold, Moisture and Remediation. These organizations would be good resources to get the most up-to-date information about mold removal and testing.

Unfortunately, people do not have control over their workplaces and buildings other than their home. This makes it even more important for someone who has mold sensitivity to keep the home safe from mold. After exposure from other sources there needs to be a safe place to go and recuperate.

For cleaning small amounts of mold in the bathroom or other areas of the home try using vinegar. Spray the vinegar on the area and let it sit for a few hours then scrub it clean. Adding an essential oil like tea tree oil, grapefruit seed extract or lavender may help cover the smell of vinegar. These different oils are antimicrobial, antibacterial and antifungal. I have read that spraying a mixture of one teaspoon tea tree oil with a cup of water will kill bathroom mold. I have tried this using both diluted tea tree oil and full strength. After using both methods, there were still signs of mold after letting it sit for a while, though some of the mold decreased when the full strength was used. Although tea tree oil did not work for the mold, I have found many other uses for it and always have a bottle handy.

Thieves Essential Oil is a product which I have not personally used but according to the research of Dr. Edward Close it is a non toxic solution for mold. Dr. Edward Close's method is to diffuse the oil for a 24 hour period into the infested building. Thieve Oil contains five essential oils: cinnamon, clove, eucalyptus, lemon and rosemary.

Another technique is spraying a food grade hydrogen peroxide mixture that is 1 part hydrogen peroxide and 2 parts water. One of my friends successfully removed mold from a trailer using this technique. He used 35% food grade hydrogen peroxide. He explained to me how the mold just dissolved and that there was just water left afterwards. Using gloves is recommending when doing this. If some hydrogen peroxide gets on the skin, the skin will turn white for a couple of hours before returning to its normal color. When cleaning with any chemical it is always a good idea to have the windows open and circulating air.

There has been some suggestion that bleach can be used to clean mold. Bleach and hydrocarbons make the organisms more mutagenic, carcinogenic and lipid soluble. (Gray, 2006, p. S152)

Molds tend to grow in dark places. Allowing the sun to come into the home during the day can help prevent it from growing. In dark areas like the basement, ultraviolet lighting may help prevent mold.

Summary of Ways to Prevent Mold

1. Replace the air conditioner filters regularly with a high rated MERV filter. Clean the drip pans.
2. Fix leaks as soon as they occur.
3. If you suspect a mold problem but can't find it, have a professional test the home.
4. Open the windows often to allow a flow of fresh air into the home.
5. Monitor indoor humidity.
6. Check window seals for cracks and condensation.
7. Properly vent appliances and rooms that produce moisture.

6 MOLD SICKNESS

Many people with mold sickness are not diagnosed correctly. Misdiagnosis occurs often since there are many other conditions that fit the profile. Additionally, there are doctors who believe that mold cannot make you sick, though that perception has been slowly changing. Many people may not even know that mold is the cause of their illness. People working in an office building that is mold contaminated may only feel ill while at work and not on the days off. For these people days off are spent recovering and the cycle restarts upon returning to work. This is often attributed to the "Monday morning blues" and not that the building they are working in is contaminated. A building is considered sick if 20% of the occupants report health symptoms while in the building and feel better upon leaving. (Esposito et al., 2014) It is not uncommon for doctors to tell their patients that their condition is related to stress from their jobs. Some of the unlucky ones will be given psychiatric drugs to handle the "stress". The people who realize that mold is an issue will have problems convincing anyone to listen. Workers in wet buildings often find themselves stone-walled when trying to convince management to fix the problems. If the building issue does get addressed, the contractor hired must know how to fix the problem or the mold will end up spreading. To correctly clean a mold infested building, techniques that are as strict as those that have been implemented for asbestos abatement should be used. If you are working in a building that has mold, it might be necessary to hire your own mold tester to see if the building was appropriately remediated. If the building management hires contractors that do not properly clean the mold, the condition in the building could worsen. I have read numerous accounts of workplaces being fixed by covering the mold with new wall board or a dropped ceiling. The problem is no longer visible to the workers but the condition still exists. Schools have often been places that may have mold issues but because of budget constraints the mold is often incorrectly remediated making the building a hazard to both the children and the employees.

For many people, exposure to mold causes some sort of discomfort. But having sensitivity to mold is a devastating issue. With each new exposure the symptoms worsen until the person becomes totally debilitated. Even if the person gets the right treatment, each subsequent exposure will still affect a mold sensitive person though the symptoms might not last as long as before treatment. The person will need to carry the right medication in case of an accidental exposure and be proactive before entering a water damaged building. Since it is impossible to know which buildings are contaminated, being proactive is not easy. Currently, this disease is a lifelong sentence. Any time a person steps into a water damaged building she/he can start to get ill within fifteen minutes. If you think of the number of buildings that you enter on any given day, how many of them have some sort of water damage? The World Health Organization (WHO) estimates that 30% of all buildings worldwide are sick buildings. (Esposito et al., 2014) Because there are a large percentage of buildings affected, making your home a safe haven does not prevent re-exposure.

What are the symptoms that someone might get when entering a water damaged building? The charts below list many of the conditions that I came across reviewing case studies. While examining the symptom chart think of how many other illnesses can be described by each symptom. This shows why it is so hard to get an accurate diagnostic. The diagnosis list makes it evident that unless the doctor really understands mold disease there is going to be a lot of needless suffering and time wasted. With mold disease time is not a friend. Each day without the correct treatment means another day of escalated immune response to mold.

Symptoms of Mold Sensitivity Syndrome

Aches	Fatigue	Pneumonia
Arthralgia	Flu like Symptoms	Rashes
Asthma	Headaches	Recurring Lyme disease
Bronchitis	Increased Urination	Respiratory issues
Concentration Problems	Low Cognitive Function	Sensitivity to temperature
Conjunctival Symptoms	Menstrual irregularities	Sinusitis
Coughing	Memory Loss	Skin sensitivity
Difficulty Focusing	Mood swings	Sleep Disturbances
Dizziness	Muscle Cramps/Spasms	Tingling
Dysosmia	Nasal Congestion/Bleeding	Tremors
Dyspnea	Nausea	Weakness
Excessive Thirst	Night Sweats	Weight gain
Eye and throat irritation	Numbness	Wheezing

Inaccurate Diagnosis for Someone with Mold Sensitivity Syndrome

Allergy	Fibromyalgia
Allergic rhinitis	Infection
Asthma	Irritable Bowel Syndrome
Attention Deficit Disorder (ADD)	Lyme disease
Chronic fatigue syndrome (CFS)	Migraine headaches
Chronic Inflammatory Response Syndrome (CIRS)	Multiple Sclerosis
	Post Traumatic Stress Disorder
Chronic Lymphocyte Leukemia	Rheumatoid arthritis
Chronic obstructive pulmonary disease (COPD)	Rhinitis
Dementia	Sarcoidosis
Depression/Mental Illness	Stress

Because of the nature of mold sensitivity disease, when treating someone with this condition, it is important to follow the correct procedure. If the person is repeatedly re-exposing themselves to a water damaged building she/he is going to continue getting ill. If a doctor realized that the person had mold sickness it would be difficult to determine which species of fungi was causing it. Most mold infested buildings have multiple biotoxins growing inside. It is not just one organism causing the inflammation, several fungi are involved. Each person with mold illness has a different combination of symptoms making it even more difficult to diagnose.

7 HUMAN BIOCHEMISTRY AND MOLD

How does a biotoxin affect one person while not causing other people to get extremely ill? In a person with a normal response to mold, the immune system responds to the toxic invasion by breaking down the biotoxin. If a person has one of the immune response genes, the HLA-DR, she/he becomes susceptible to the neurotoxin associated with that particular gene. The human leukocyte antigen (HLA) molecules are antigens that determine how our bodies respond to stimulus. People with the worst mold illness have the HLA-DR types of 11-3-52B or 12-3-52B with genotype 4-3-53. These types are passed down from our ancestors. If one person in the family has one of these genes it would be a good idea to get the rest of the family members tested to be able to implement a game plan. 11-3-52B and 4-3-53 are also seen in people with Lyme disease. An interesting physical characteristic of people with the mold gene is the person's wingspan is longer than their height.

If the immune response does not get triggered, the biotoxins remain in the body and are able to cause severe damage. These free circulating toxins bind to the surface of toll receptors (proteins that have a role in the innate immune system) and other receptors causing inflammation by producing cytokines (small proteins that affect cell behavior), activation of the complement system (part of the immune system that helps the body clear pathogens) and transforming growth factor (TGF) Beta-1. Nerve function is also affected by biotoxins.

High levels of cytokines cause unwanted negative effects in the body. The first is the release of matrix metallopeptidase 9 (MMP-9) (enzyme that is encoded by the MMP9 gene). Excess MMP-9 causes inflammation to soft tissue. High doses of MMP-9 have been found in people with breast cancer. (Lin et al., 2014) MMP-9 combines with plasminogen activator inhibitor-1 (PAI-1) causing blood clots and blocked arteries. The Cytokines also increase levels of PA1-1. High cytokine levels decrease blood flow which means less endothelial growth factor (VEGF) reaches the tissues. VEGF is a signal protein that is part of the system that brings homeostasis to the tissues when the oxygen supply is low from inadequate blood circulation. Since VEGF does not reach the tissues it will cause fatigue, muscle cramps and difficulty breathing. An increase in cytokines will also cause people with certain HLA genotypes to produce antibodies to gliadin (gluten protein component), actin (multi-functional protein that forms microfilaments), anti-neutrophil cytoplasmic antibody (ANCA), cardiolipins (common membrane protein) and many others. This results in the body treating things that are normal as foreigners and trying to get rid of them. High levels of complement C4-A (C4-A) (C4-A is a protein) get produced when there are high levels of cytokine. Once C4-A is turned on, it continually gets activated resulting in always having low oxygen in the tissues. High C4-A is also associated with rashes and muscle spasms. Cytokines will bind with leptin receptors in the hypothalamus which blocks the production of alpha melanocyte stimulating hormone (MSH). Leptin is the hormone that is associated with satiety. It is made by the fat cells and regulates how much fat is stored in the body. Leptin is responsible for signaling the body that it is time to stop eating. MSH influences skin pigmentation and concentration.

MSH deficiency causes headaches, muscle fatigue, unstable body temperature and difficulty concentrating. When MSH is low, melatonin production also gets reduced. Melatonin is responsible for sleep. Low MSH results in chronic and usual pain by lowering endorphin. The main function of endorphins is to inhibit pain. Malabsorption of food in the gut is caused by low MSH. White blood cells eventually don't function right which allows infections to easily invade the body. If MSH is low, multiple antibiotic resistant coagulase negative staphylococci (MARCoNS) are allowed to survive in mucous membranes causing biofilms. Staph causes a further reduction of MSH. This downward spiral has many negative consequences for the person invaded by biotoxins. Low MSH decreases the production of anti-diuretic hormone (ADH) which is made in the pituitary gland. ADH is also known as vasopressin. Decreased ADH causes frequent urination, low blood serum levels, excessive thirst and static electricity. In the beginning stages of mold illness the cortisol (a steroid hormone) and adrenocorticotropic hormone (ACTH) may be high but as the illness progresses the levels drop to low or bottom of the normal range. Cortisol is the hormone associated with stress and low levels of blood glucose. Elevated cortisol levels lead to proteolysis and muscle wasting. Cushing syndrome is associated with hypercortisolism. Addison's disease and Nelson's syndrome are associated with hypocortisolism. ACTH is also known as corticotropin. Its production is often related to stress. Elevated ACTH is associated with Cushing's disease while deficiency is related to adrenal insufficiency. In many organisms ACTH is related to circadian rhythm. Just looking at the cortisol and ACTH lab results you can see why getting an accurate diagnose for mold disease is so difficult.

Vasoactive intestinal polypeptide (VIP) plays a similar role to MSH in regulating inflammatory responses. VIP deficiency is an important piece in understanding mold illness. When VEGF and VIP are low, oxygen does not get delivered to the capillary beds causing shortness of breath. VIP is an important factor for cellular communication that is tied to cyclic adenosine monophosphate (cAMP). cAMP is derived from adenosine triphosphate (ATP) and is used for intracellular signal transduction (activation of a specific receptor located on the cell or inside the cell which triggers a biochemical response). A defect in this regulation can cause problems in almost every cell. cAMP helps hormones like glucagon and adrenaline pass through the cell membrane. It activates protein kinase. Protein kinase is an enzyme that modifies other proteins. VIP will determine which messages get inside the cell, thus in effect controlling the cell.

When biotoxins are in the body the results of blood tests rarely show issues with blood count or metabolic profiles. The only exception is abnormal liver levels caused by bile flow stoppage. This stoppage is related to a decrease in the gamma-glutamyl transpeptidase (GGTP) enzyme which is an important enzyme for bile flow. GGTP is found in many tissues especially the liver. Elevated levels are associated with liver, biliary and pancreas diseases. Low levels are associated with high triglycerides, hypothyroidism, hypothalamic malfunction and low levels of serum magnesium.

Another effect of the leptin receptors being blocked is an increase of leptin in the blood stream. This is why people with mold disease tend to have high leptin levels. The body's inability to utilize leptin leads to the loss of the ability to suppress appetite which results in weight gain.

There is a specific mycotoxin, Satratoxin H, which affects the nervous system in a different way. Satratoxin H actually initiates apoptosis in nerve cells which leads to their death. Since the primary function of the nervous system is carrying messages within the body, death of nerve cells causes an extremely negative impact on the body's ability to send messages. (Karunasena, Larrañaga, Simoni, Douglas, & Straus, 2010)

Endocrine disruption can cause a host of issues. A study was done to determine if the mycotoxin Ochratoxin A was an endocrine disruptor. The conclusion was that the steroid receptors were not affected but it had a potential to cause endocrine disruption by interfering with steroidogenesis. The proper function of adrenal glands, testes and ovaries depend on the steroidogenesis pathway, the role of which is vital to human health and development. (Frizzell, Verhaegen, Ropstad, Elliott, & Connolly, 2013)

Reduction in cognitive function is a symptom associated with people who have mold sensitivity syndrome. Until recently there was no way to determine how the inflammation from mold caused inflammation in the brain leading to reduction in cognition. TGF beta-1 and IL-1B are elevated in people with inflammatory response to mold. Both TGF beta-1 and IL-1B play a role in loosening the tight junctions in the blood brain barrier. A new technique is in the works for testing the brain to understand the effects of mold on it. A computer program called NeuroQuant® has been used for people with traumatic brain injury for several years. This program measures the brain volumes from an accurate magnetic resonance imaging (MRI) scan in fifteen different areas. Dr. David E. Ross has been using this program on his mold patients. The preliminary results show a unique white matter fingerprint and injury in the caudate nucleus of the gray matter structure. The preliminary data has already shown the link between cognitive decline and mold. This new technique looks promising as a new diagnostic tool for mold sensitivity. (Shoemaker, 2010-2013; http://vaneuropsychiatry.org/)

A healthy mitochondria is required for proper cell functioning and energy. The mold can damage the mitochondria causing DNA mutations and a reduction in ATP. Inadequate levels of ATP can cause fatigue.

The physiology and function of the following pillars of Functional Medicine -- assimilation, defense and repair -- are affected by fungi. The intestinal tract becomes weakened by excess fungi. The person is also more prone to infection and respiratory issues. This can be caused by the breathing and ingestion of mold. People lacking the gene that triggers the immune response to create antibodies against the mold will have mold issues forever since the liver will never get the signal to break the fungi down. Without the defense and repair triggered, the person has no way to overcome the illness.

With a mold sensitive person the biotransformation and elimination routes stop functioning accurately from the overload of constant exposure to hidden sources of mold.

The Functional Medicine transport system is concerned with the distribution of substances to the appropriate sites within the body. This system is affected in mold sensitive people. There is an excess of MMP-9 which causes inflammation to soft tissue affecting structural integrity. Transport is also affected by blood clots and blocked arteries which occur when MMP-9 combines with PAI-1. Restricted blood flow and reduced oxygen levels reach the tissues because of high cytokine levels in the capillaries attracting white blood cells. The result is a reduction in VEGF. Low levels of VEGF cause fatigue, muscle cramps and shortness of breath.

An environmental antecedent that would affect someone with mold sensitivity is a drought. People with mold sensitivity tend to be thirsty when water is not available as there is a negative impact on all of the body's functions. Since people with mold sensitivity tend to give more electrical shocks, walking on a carpeted floor will trigger greater static electricity. Though these things are not directly related to mold they are part of the makeup of someone with the issue.

(http://betterhealthguy.com/joomla/blog/251-biotoxin-illness-conference-2011; Brennan & Mantzoros, 2006; Friedman & Halaas, 1998; http://www.survivingmold.com/diagnosis/the-biotoxin-pathway)

8 IMPACT ON SOCIETY

In recent years there have been lots of major rain storms causing massive water damage to buildings. After Hurricane Katrina, toxic black mold, Stachybotrys chartarum and Penicillium mold could be found in the water damaged homes. Black mold has cytotoxic macrocyclic trichothecene mycotoxins which inhibits protein synthesis which is why it is a hazardous to one's health.

Besides the two molds listed above there are other toxic molds that can be found in buildings. There is a list of various molds and toxic components at the end of this chapter.

To clean a water damaged building requires knowledge not only about building structures but about conditions that allow fungus to grow and spread. Without the proper removal, the fungus can grow rapidly. As mentioned earlier, new fungus is growing every thirty minutes. If part of the clean-up includes paints containing benomyl the building can end up with mutated fungus everywhere. Even a person who does not have a mold sensitive genotype can be affected by daily breathing mold substances. Unfortunately, properly fixing the problem is costly. It can sometimes take years to identify a leak and while the investigation is going on, fungus continually grows. Destroying buildings with a mold issue is quite expensive. Often times the issue comes down to what do you want the government to spend money on, fixing buildings or educating children?

There has been a lot of litigation due to water damaged buildings. Cases cost a lot of money to pursue. The sick person who is already spending a lot on health care is fighting against a corporation or a government that has the resources and energy to fight these cases. Many of the cases in the past were lost due to lack of scientific evidence. As more scientific evidence becomes available linking health issues to mold, the courts will have to take a different stance. In March 2012, the courts in New York overturned the Manhattan appellate court's decision which disallowed people from making claims related to health from living in a moldy building. In 2011, New York had 15,942 violations issued by housing inspectors for mold-related conditions. After Hurricane Sandy, the number of mold violations probably increased. In New York, if the landlord paints over the mold, the violation is closed. Painting over mold does not stop mold from reproducing and causing problems.

When your health is compromised dealing with the additional burden of proving the leaky building caused your illness is not the first thing on your mind. Unless the public at large becomes more educated on mold related illness, the problem with water damaged buildings will persist. With an educated public, the government will be forced to enact some measures to protect the people especially our children.

Many children are attending schools that contain mold. Moldy buildings reduce the ability to be focused and learn. What will these children do as adults if the places that they were sent to learn were not conducive to that activity?

Addressing the mold problem provides the opportunity for new innovations. This can stimulate the economy. There is one new invention that shows promise in helping water damaged buildings. The product was designed by an Austrian engineer name Wilhelm Mohorn. The design is a new technique for drying a building that requires less of the mold damaged building to be destroyed. Currently, it is sold in Switzerland, the United Kingdom and Italy by the Aquapol Company.

Since mold sensitivity syndrome is very complex it gives scientists an opportunity to learn more about how the body works with all its pieces. Any new discoveries can help solve the challenges of other diseases in addition to mold illness.

(http://www.aquapol.co.uk/index.php?go=company/history; Ebbehøj et al., 2005; Meklin et al., 2002; Meklin et al., 2003; Meklin et al., 2005; Savilahti, Uitti, Laippala, Husman, & Roto, 2000; Savilahti, Uitti, Roto, Laippala, & Husman, 2001; Scheel, Rosing, & Farone, 2001; Vesley, 2012; Wålinder et al., 2001; Yang, Chiu, Chiu, & Kao, 1997)

Types of Molds and Toxic Components

Name	Toxin	
Alternaria tenuissima species	Alternariols Altertoxin I Number of unknown metabolites	Tentoxin Tenuazonic acids
Aspergillus flavus	3-nitropropionic acid Aflatoxin B$_1$ Aspergillic acid	Cyclopiazonic acid Metabolites kojic acid
Aspergillus fumigatus	Fumigaclavines Fumitoxins Fumitremorgens	Gliotoxins Tryptoquivalins, Verruculogen
Aspergillus niger	Ochratoxin A	
Aspergillus ochraceus	Ochratoxin A Penicillic acid Viomellein	Vioxanthin Xanthomegnin
Aspergillus ustus	Austalides Carcinogenic austocystins	Toxic austamides Toxic austdiols Versicolorin C
Aspergillus versicolor	Carcinogenic mycotoxin sterigmatocystin and related compounds	
Chaetomium globosum	Cytotoxic chaetomins and chaetoglobosins (inhibitor of cell division and glucose transport) Sterigmatocystins	
Memnoniella echinata	Components related to mycophenolic acid Dechlorogriseofulvins Griseofulvin	Spirocyclic drimanes Trichodermin Trichodermol
Penicillium brevicompactum	Asperphenamate Botryodiploidin Brevianamides	Mycophenolic acid Raistrick phenols
Penicillium chrysogenum	Secalonic acid D	
Penicillium expansum	Citrinin Chaetoglobosins Communesins	Patulin Roquefortine C
Penicillium polonicum	3-methoxy-viridicatin Anacine Cyclopenins Cytotoxic penicillic acid Nephrotoxic glycopeptides (causing Balkan nephropathy endemic)	Tremorgenic verrucosidins Verrucofortine Verrucosidin Viridicatins
Stachybotrys chartarum	Cytotoxic macrocyclic trichothecenes (inhibit protein synthesis) Roridin E	Satratoxin Verrucarin
Trichoderma	Acetyl ester trichodermin Cytotoxic proteins (these inactivate ribosomes) Gliotoxin Harzianum A Numerous low molecular weight metabolites	Peptaibols Viridin Volatile lactones Volatile pyrones Trichothecenes Trichodermol

(Nielsen, 2003)

9 INCIDENCE AND PREVALENCE

It is hard to determine what percentage of the population actually has mold sensitivity syndrome or how many buildings are actually damaged. The World Health Organization has estimated that 30% of all buildings worldwide have a problem. With recent heavy rainfall and flooding this number may have increased. Many people that have an issue with mold sensitivity have been misdiagnosed. Others do not realize that a building is causing them any harm.

There is enough evidence that shows being in a water damaged building causes health issues. Looking at the number of studies done around the world, this issue happens quite often. In a study of daycare workers in damp and moldy buildings in Taipei, the study concluded that people who work in damp moldy buildings have a statistically significant prevalence of Sick Building Syndrome. A study in Taiwan measured the relationship of children living in damp homes and respiratory symptoms. The conclusion from this study was that respiratory issues were higher in damp homes than in non damp ones.

A cross sectional study conducted in Finland determined that children attending school with moisture damage were more likely to have infections and had antibiotics more often than other children. In this study when the school remediated the problem, the children's health issues were no longer a problem. Another studied found that when children are exposed in school to molds, solvents, and plasticizers, they had higher rates of asthma and nighttime breathlessness.

A study of Finish office workers determined that adults were nine-times as likely to get adult-onset asthma working in a building that had damp floor coverings than workers in the same field not working under such conditions. A hospital in Montana with water damage found that workers had less respiratory symptoms when they were away from work.

A water damaged school building in New Orleans determined that employees had more rashes, nasal and lower respiratory symptoms than the comparison school.

This small sampling of studies is just a taste of how many people are being exposed on a daily basis to water damaged buildings with resultant health issues.

(Kim et al., 2007; Li, Hsu, & Lu, 1997; Rao, Cox-Ganser, Chew, Doekes, & White, 2005; Savilahti et al., 2000; Thomas, Burton, Mueller, Page, & Vesper, 2012; Tuomainen, Seuri, & Sieppi, 2004; Yang et al., 1997)

10 CURRENT MEDICAL APPROACHES

Unfortunately, many of the people that have mold sensitivity syndrome are not treated for that disease. There are many doctors that do not believe that people can get sick from mold. Since they do not understand that people get sick from mold, any medical tests that are given usually bear no relevance to the disease. At the present time, there is no conventional treatment for mold sensitivity syndrome. Most people are treated for the other symptoms that they have. Treating a person with mold sensitivity syndrome in the wrong manner causes additional problems for that person.

While taking the client's oral history any comments from the client about mold exposure are often ignored. The doctor will proceed to take all the wrong blood tests which return normal results. It is very rare for the blood count or metabolic profiles to be abnormal in a person with mold illness. When the amount of the total oxygen is taken in the blood sample it does not reflect the oxygen levels in the capillaries.

Another test that a conventional doctor might give their mold sick patient is a pulmonary stress test. Since the cells are oxygen deprived, taking this test will give erroneous results making it appear as if the person has heart problems.

If the person is tested for Lyme disease and has the HLA types of 11-3-52B and 4-3-53, she/he may be needlessly treated for Lyme disease when she/he has mold illness.

Some doctors may prescribe Prednisone to their patients due to their symptoms. This may treat the symptoms but it does nothing to kill the fungus that the person has in their body. It definitely does not address the re-exposure. Prednisone is known to lower ACTH. Because people with mold sensitivity syndrome have reduced MSH, the cortisol and ACTH will be higher in the earlier stages of the illness and then drop to low levels. In some cases the person may get treated for leaky gut. This symptom is caused by low MSH that results in diarrhea from malabsorption in the gut.

Since there is weight gain caused by the leptin receptors being blocked, doctors may prescribe exercise and/or diet for the patient. The weight cannot be controlled with exercise or diet. Exercise is a difficult task for people with mold illness because of inadequate oxygen delivery to the tissues both during and after exercise. Oxygen is required for the cells to prevent inflammation and allow normal functioning. Since oxygen levels are already low, any kind of aerobic exercise is only going to cause more inflammation and pain to a person with mold disease. "VO2 Max" is a test that measures the amount of oxygen that your body utilizes during exercise. If the "VO2 Max" test is given and the results are low, the person will be told that she/he is not exercising. If the person attempts to exercise his/her health will spiral downward.

Some people may have surgery to correct nose bleed problems. For most people the way that mold enters the body is through inhalation. Since mold is inhaled, unless a person that is sensitive to mold no longer enters a water damaged building, problems with nose bleeds will persist.

Many people with mold illness are referred by their doctor to a specialist. They may get bounced around many times without getting any answers as to what is causing their sickness. After exhausting many doctors often it is decided the there is nothing wrong with the person, it is all in her/his head and now it's off to a Psychiatrist.

Until the disease is recognized as a viable disease the current testing approach is only going to cause misdiagnosis and lost time for the person as she/he becomes increasingly ill with each new exposure. In the end no matter what intervention the doctor tries unless the person is removed from the mold condition he/she will remain sick. With each passing day that the real cause of illness is not addressed, the person gets sicker and sicker by returning to an environment that made him/her ill in the first place.

11 FUNCTIONAL MEDICINE APPROACH

The Functional Medicine approach is based on forming a partnership with the patient. All the information is gathered and the patient is given the time to tell his/her story. By carefully listening to the story, evaluating intake forms, and ordering any necessary tests, the practitioner can determine what antecedents, triggers, and mediators are involved with the condition. Antecedents are the predisposing factors that contribute to a condition. There are a few antecedents for a person that has mold disease. There are certain genes that predispose a person to this condition: 11-3-52B and 4-3-53 or 12-3-52B and 4-3-53. The 4-3-53 genotype subtypes of 0401, 0402 and 0404 are the worst ones to have if a person is exposed to mold. Having long arms in comparison to height is another factor for people with this disease. Exposure to mold even for a short time in one's lifetime predisposes the person with the mold gene combination to becomes ill. Exposure to other environmental toxins can exacerbate the situation. Medications like prednisone are also antecedents.

Triggers are events that cause the condition to occur. Any time a person is exposed to mold, the condition is triggered. When a person enters a building with water damage or is near a field that was once sprayed with Benlate an immune response occurs.

Mediators are the perpetuating factors that contribute to the condition. Contributing factors are dieting, aerobic exercise, improperly cleaned moldy buildings, and incorrect diagnosis.

Unfortunately, unless a person lives inside a bubble there is not much that one can do to prevent himself/herself from ever entering a water damaged building. People working in certain professions, like plumbers and construction workers may have an occupational hazard due to the increased likelihood of being exposed to mold. Searching in PubMed, I was unable to find any clinical trials to support this assumption.

Using a timeline is a helpful tool especially for a person with a mold condition. By plotting the occurrences of illness that negatively impact health across a timeline, it may be possible to identify buildings that have mold conditions and avoid those buildings.

Approaching the condition of mold sensitivity has to be done in a specific manner. The first step is proper screening. This can be done ahead of time by having the person fill out a comprehensive questionnaire. If the person has non resolving respiratory issues, autoimmune disease or frequent headaches, even if water damage was not identified during the initial question screening mold may be the culprit. The presence of hidden mold can be the cause of the person's sickness; in many instances the person may be unaware of his/her exposure to mold. As indicated in *"Symptoms of Mold Sensitivity Syndrome"* and *"Inaccurate Diagnosis for Someone with Mold Sensitivity Syndrome"* charts mold disease can be diagnosed as many different diseases.

Below is a sampling of items that should be considered during an initial screening. Below is a sampling of items that should be considered during an initial screening. Free checklists can be found at healthwright.info. These can be helpful to bring with you to doctor's appointments.

Questions Concerning Biotoxin Exposure

Anthrax Vaccination	High Speed (over 25 mph) Vehicle Crash
Building with Odors	Ill After Eating Fish
Building Occupant Consider Sick	In Ocean During Red Tide
Contact Blue-Green Algae	Leaks in Home
Contact Fish Kill	Lion Fish Sting
Contact Fungus	Other Biotoxins
Contact Inland Lakes	Persian Gulf War
Contact Non-Ocean Coastal Waters	Spider Bite
Contact Poisonous Organism	Tick Bites (to rule out Lyme)
Exposure to Fungus	Unexplained Rashes
Farming Land Abandoned for Re-cropping Problems	Warped wood floor boards in home
Flooding in home	Yellow Rain in South East Asia
Front Loading machine used	

(http://www.survivingmold.com/diagnosis/the-biotoxin-pathway)

Questions Concerning Occupational Exposure or Heavy Metal Exposure

9/11	Organic Solvents
Lead	Pesticides
Mercury	Persistent Organo-Chlorine Compounds
Other Metals	Petroleum Products
Other Neurotoxic Compounds	

Questions Concerning Current Illness

Attention Deficit Hyperactivity Disorder
Autism
Bacteria
Bell's Palsy
Biotoxin Exposure Related Illness
Brown Recluse (or other poisonous) Spider
Bite
Charcot Marie Tooth Syndrome
Chemical Sensitivity
Chronic Fatigue
Chronic Soft Tissue Injury
Ciguatera Seafood Poisoning

Depression
Fibromyalgia
Fungus or Mycotoxicosis
Gulf War Syndrome
Irritable Bowel Syndrome
Learning Disability
Lion Fish Sting
Pfiesteria (Possible Estuary Associated Syndrome)
Sick Building Syndrome
Sensory Neural Hearing Loss
Tick borne illness/Lyme Disease

(http://www.survivingmold.com/diagnosis/the-biotoxin-pathway)

Questions Concerning Diagnosed Illnesses

Addison's disease
Alzheimer's disease
Allergy
Amyotrophic Lateral Sclerosis (ALS)
Another Condition Involving Neurologic
Function
Asthma
Attention Deficit Disorder
Chronic obstructive pulmonary disease (COPD)
Cushing syndrome

Diabetes
Fibromyalgia
Low Vision or Blindness
Lyme disease
Multiple Sclerosis
Nelson's syndrome
Ocular Disease (e.g., cataract)
Parkinson's Disease
Post Traumatic Stress Disorder
Retinal Disease (e.g., glaucoma)

(http://www.survivingmold.com/diagnosis/the-biotoxin-pathway)

Questions Concerning Lifestyle

Air purifier or water filters – last time changed filter – type filter used
Acrylic fingernails
Aerosol sprays used like hair spray
Carpeted home
Central air conditioner
Dental cavities

Dry cleaning
Exterminator
Fabric softeners
Hair coloring
Pesticides
Pets
Scented soaps, detergents, potpourri, perfumes

(http://www.survivingmold.com/diagnosis/the-biotoxin-pathway)

Rating Questions Concerning Degree of Symptoms

Abdominal Pain
Bright Light Sensitivity
Confusion
Cough
Depression
Diarrhea
Disorientation
Dizzy After Standing
Fatigue

Headache
Joint Pain
Memory Loss
Metallic Taste
Muscle Ache
Muscle Cramp
Other
Red Eyes
Reduced Concentration

Short of Breath
Sinus Congestion
Skin Pain
Tearing
Tingling
Vertigo
Weakness

(http://www.survivingmold.com/diagnosis/the-biotoxin-pathway)

Visual contrast sensitivity (VCS) test can be taken, if the results of the screening questionnaire indicate that the person has been exposed to any biotoxins. The VCS assessment is useful for early detection of neurotoxins and disruption in neurological function. By measuring visual functioning, this test determines if the toxins have any effect on the visual system. The retina of the eye is less protected than the brain from toxin exposures. In order to take the test each eye individually needs to be corrected to 20:50 or 20:20 with glasses. The test does not work if the eyesight is not correct. With VCS five spatial frequencies from small to large lines appear in different directions on the computer monitor. The frequencies are associated with different physiologic processes. Studies have shown that the spatial frequency of visual contrast in people that have been exposed to toxins is deficient in the mid, mid-to-high and mid-to-low areas. The person taking the test determines the direction of different lines. Because of the test design it is difficult to get false positives. I took the test and got positive results. Given my exposure history and my reaction to mold the results did not surprise me. The VCS screening allows for early diagnosis. After a positive VCS treatment can be started while waiting for lab results. Follow-up VCS tests help determine if the treatment has been working. VCS has shown improvements on retests with the correct treatment. Dr. Ritchie Shoemaker has seen clinically that 92% of people with biotoxins illness will get a positive VCS result. Rarely, there are false negative results. (Hudnell, House, & Shoemaker, 2003; Shoemaker, 2009; Shoemaker, 2010)

Lab tests can help a Doctor confirm diagnosis and track the success of the disease intervention protocol.

Suggested Labs Tests

ACTH
Aerobic culture (nasal)
Androstenedione
Anti-cardiolipin antibodies IgA, IgM, IgG SST
Anti-nuclear antibody
Anti-diuretic hormone (ADH)
C-reactive protein (semi-quantitative)
Cortisol
Dehydroepiandrosterone sulfate
GGT
Fungal Identification (FID) Profile
HLA-DR by PCR
ICAT (Allergy Testing) Profile

Interleukin 1-beta
Leptin
Matrix metalloproteinase-9
MSH
Myco- M7 Series Mycotoxin Profile
Mycobacterium Identification (MB) Panel
Osmolality
Plasminogen activator inhibitor
Prolactin
Reverse T3 (RT3)
Testosterone
Thyroid stimulating hormone (TSH)
Thyroxine (T4)
TNF alpha

(D. Haase, February 12, 2013; http://www.survivingmold.com/diagnosis/the-biotoxin-pathway)

Labs Tests - Specimen used by Dr. Shoemaker

ACTH
Aerobic Culture-Nasal
ANA
Androstenedione
Anti-Diuretic Hormone
Anticardiolipin Ab's
Cardio CRP (hs)
Cortisol

DHEA, Sulfate
GGT
HLA
ILB-1
Insulin
Leptin Level
MMP-9
MSH

PAI-1 Activity
Prolactin Level
Serum Osmolality
T4
TNF Alpha
Total Testosterone
TSH

(http://www.survivingmold.com/diagnosis/the-biotoxin-pathway)

Specific Labs Results to Watch For

Low	High	Genotype
ACTH	C4-A	4-3-53 worst subtypes 0401, 0402 and 0404
Cortisol	Leptin	HLA 11-3-52B
MSH	MMP-9	
VEGF	Reverse T3	
VIP	TGF beta-1	

(D. Haase, February 12, 2013; http://www.survivingmold.com/diagnosis/the-biotoxin-pathway)

The normal reference range for MSH is 35-81. Some labs have lowered this number to be 0-40. When questioned about why the labs changed this range, the response was that more patients were showing in the lower range so it must be the normal one. This appears to be a misguided justification since the very fact that the patients are looking for treatment to a health problem would preclude them from being considered normal.

Once the person has been identified as having mold sensitivity syndrome, there are some steps that can be taken to improve his/her health. The most important and first step is to remove the source of the problem. If the source of the mold is in your home, this will mean hiring a contractor that is knowledgeable in mold removal and environmental health. Removing mold by one's self is not advised unless one is trained in that area. There are many places that can be missed during the clean up process and for someone with this condition any mold left behind poses a threat. Also the overexposure to mold during self removal could cause the condition to escalate to a much worse state than is already occurring.

Places often missed during this process are small holes in pipes leaking behind dry wall. Underneath the refrigerator and dishwasher, water from condensation can leak on the floor causing mold. Front load washing machines will get moldy if the door is closed before all the water dries inside the washer.

Make sure the humidity level in the building does not exceed sixty percent. Dirt floors in basements are another source of mold contamination. Unwanted infestation in a home from termites and carpenter ants can bring moisture into a home. The wooden mulch put in the garden around the outside of the house to keep the soil moist is another source of mold. All mulch should be removed. It can be replaced with river rock. It is important that the plants and trees around the house allow free air to circulate. Large trees that are close to the house can block some of the air flow into the house. Keeping the trees trimmed and branches off of the house will help with this problem.

Mold can grow underneath carpets as a result of liquid spills. Mold is not the only issue with carpets. They also attract dirt, as well as toxic, and non-toxic chemicals. All carpets need to be removed and replaced with either tiles or hardwood floors. There is a good chance that mold will be noticed under the carpet during the removal process. (Crinnion, 2010)

After the mold has been removed the surfaces can be painted. Using a paint with low VOX is better for ones overall health. Never paint over a moldy surface to cover it. The mold will still continue to grow under the painted surface.

Finding all the potential hazard sources in the home takes good detective work. Any contaminated items that cannot be cleaned need to be thrown away. Places that were missed during the removal process pose a continual health threat.

Once your home has been made safe, clean up any leaks or floods as soon as possible within the first forty-eight hours to prevent any mold from forming. Tea tree oil makes a good cleaner to fight mold due to its antimicrobial activity. The newly contaminated surfaces can be scrubbed with a tea tree and water solution. Fruit with thick non edible peels can also be cleaned with tea tree oil as a protection against fungi. (Cháfer, Sánchez-González, González-Martínez, & Chiralt, 2012; Forrer, Kulik, Filippi, & Waltimo, 2013)

The car is another place that may require mold removal. Rain water on shoes and from open doors can get into the car. If the car does not have the proper air circulation to dry the water, mold will form. If possible leave the windows open after a rainstorm to air the car out.

If the source of contamination is one's place of employment expect an uphill battle with the company to get it fixed. Do your own ERMI testing once the job is completed to make sure that the building is safe for your reentry. The ERMI results should not exceed two and for some people one is all that they can tolerate. The other thing to consider is looking for another job or requesting a transfer to another building if the company has multiple locations.

Once the person has been identified as having biotoxins, treatment can start. There is no need to wait until the mold condition has been removed. The biotoxins that are in the body need to be removed. The stool is one of the routes of elimination that works well for this purpose. Prescription Cholestyramine or over the counter supplement butyrate have both been shown to be effective for this purpose.

Cholestyramine is a cholesterol binding drug that can bind to the toxins from the bile preventing reabsorption. This drug comes in powder form. One scoop four times a day can be added to eight ounces of apple juice or distilled water. A half hour after taking the Cholestyramine drink, eat some form of healthy fat. This helps push the toxins out of the bile and into the gut where the Cholestyramine can absorb them. One of the known side effects with Cholestyramine is constipation. Drinking plenty of water and eating foods that are high in fiber helps keep the bowels moving. Eating fruits like figs, apricots, papaya, peaches, pears, and vegetables like cauliflower, broccoli, Brussels sprouts, carrots, green beans, and peas are sources of extra fiber. People have experienced positive results within a month of taking Cholestyramine. Cholestyramine is usually taken for 2-4 weeks. The length of time on the medication will depend on when the VCS normalizes.

Butyrate is a short 4-carbon chain fatty acid that is known to mobilize fats, clearing biotoxins and lowering TNF-a. Butyrate is a histone deacetylase inhibitor which means it regulates histones. Histones are chromatin proteins that regulate DNA copying. Butyrate inhibits one of the enzymes that cause changes in the DNA. The suggested daily dosage for an adult is 500 to 2000 mg. (Fusunyan, Quinn, Ohno, MacDermott, & Sanderson, 1998; Speight, 2006)

When taking either Cholestyramine or butyrate, it is advisable to also take a good fatty acid that is a combination of omega-3, 6 and 9 or good quality fish oil. This will quench the cell membranes to enable them to work well. One brand that makes the omega 3-6-9 blend is Udo's Choice. There are many companies that make good quality fish oil: Vital Choice, Green Pasture and Carlson to name a few.

Food choices are another consideration. Foods like blue cheese that contain fungi should be avoided. Gluten should be completely removed from the diet for three or four months especially for those people with positive anti-gliadin antibodies and for people with high MMP-9. People with high MMP-9 should consume a no-amylose diet. Foods that are high in amylose spike the blood sugar levels promoting resistance to insulin and leptin. Avoidance of all sugars and grains is part of the no amylose diet. Root vegetables like yams, carrots and potatoes also need to be avoided. Just about all fruit except bananas, along with lean meats and green vegetables are permitted. The no-amylose diet also works for people who are at risk for obesity and insulin resistant diabetes. (Shoemaker, 2005)

In general anyone with a mold condition should avoid all sugar. Molds thrive on sugar. In order to ensure freshness of food, it is better to buy it in small quantities rather than large ones which will not be used for awhile. This will help prevent the potential of mold developing on the food. Since the mold is not visible to the naked eye until colonies are formed this will prevent consumption of food that has a little mold contamination. Eating a healthy diet with lots of dark leafy greens and few processed foods will help the bodies' ability to detoxify. Members of the brassicas from the cruciferae family which include broccoli, cauliflower, Brussels sprouts, kale, and cabbage are helpful for detoxification. Increasing the amount of fiber in the diet will help normalize the bowel function.

Eating organic foods as much as possible to prevent an additional burden of pesticides will help the body so it is not trying to detoxify too many things. The Environmental Working Group has a list of the most sprayed foods known as the "Dirty Dozen" and the least sprayed foods "Clean 15" that are available from the website: http://www.ewg.org. There is also an application that can be downloaded to the phone, so the list is at your fingertips while in the supermarket.

Seafood can also pose a problem. Large carnivorous fish like swordfish, shark, tuna, and halibut are high in mercury. Farmed fish are not a better option because they contain high levels of polychlorinated biphenyls (PCBs) from their diet. Meat that is not organic is another source of persistent pollutants.

Avoiding foods that one is sensitive to can help reduce the immunological response. Getting a serum blood test which tests both allergy and sensitivity or doing an elimination diet can help identify those foods. Eliminating the foods that are offensive to the body will help the person feel better usually within three or four days. To do the elimination diet, start by keeping a food journal for at least a week, then determine which foods are eaten most often and which foods you crave. Use those foods as the basis for the elimination process. For the next three to six weeks completely eliminate the food from your diet. You can choose multiple foods to eliminate or start with one at a time. When eliminating multiple foods it is best to reintroduce them one at a time over a three day period. If you have any negative reactions to the food completely remove it from the diet. Once you have been healing for awhile and feel strong you can try the eliminated foods again. If you are eating processed foods, check the labels carefully to make sure the product does not contain any traces of the eliminated foods.

Partial List of Fungal Mold Containing Foods

Aged Cheese	Fruit Juice	Sauerkraut
Alcohol -Especially Dark Beer	Mushrooms	Sorghum
Barley	Old Leftovers	Strawberries
Bread	Peanuts	Tomato products
Corn	Processed Meats	Wheat
Cottonseed Oil	Raspberries	Wine (fungi is used in
Dried Fruit	Rye	fermentation process)

Staph growth (MARCoNS) creates biofilm in the deepest part of the nose. Biofilm is a group of microorganisms that have joined together to form a matrix. The biofilm must be broken in order for the person to recover. The biofilm also acts as a protective mechanism against antibiotics. Nasal sprays can break down biofilm. The sprays often used are either colloidal silver or prescription BEG spray (contains Bactroban, EDTA and gentamicin). EDTA is the active ingredient in BEG spray that breaks down the biofilm. BEG spray may cause side effects of kidney problems, nerve damage, hearing loss and balance problems. The sprays are used twice a day for several months. Be sure to discuss the pros and cons of each technique with your doctor.

Once the MARCoNS are negative, VCS is negative and the ERMI is < 2 a nasal spray of vasoactive intestinal polypeptide (VIP) can be used. VIP has the added benefit of reducing C4-A, restoring neuropeptide inflammation control, correcting secondary hormonal issues, lowering TGF Beta-1, raising VEGF and raising MSH. VIP is only effective if there is no source of mold exposure. (Monteiro et al., 2012; Shoemaker, 2010, p. 398-399)

Some people have used Neti Pots to clean the nasal cavity. I have tried this and ended up with a massive headache. I probably did not use it correctly. If it is not used correctly the biofilm could potentially be uprooted and moved to another location in the body. Since the nasal cavity is near the brain, I would be concerned about pushing the toxins into the brain. If you have a lot of experience with the Neti Pot just bear in mind if you get any headaches or other new symptoms after its use, stop using it.

Dave Asprey, founder of The Bulletproof Executive successfully alternated twice daily between a silver nasal spray and diluted iodine solution wash to help his mold related sinus problem. To wash using the iodine solution he put iodine solution in a bowl, his face was placed inside the bowl and he breathed the solution through the nose while tilting the head backwards from side to side cleaning the sinuses and eventually allowing the solution to leave through the mouth. I personally would put the solution in a spray bottle and spray some in the nasal cavity. Alternating the different types of solutions between days will keep the MARCoNS off guard and less likely to become resistant to the breakup of their colony. 3% food grade hydrogen peroxide or ozonated water with salt are other substances that can also be used to cleanse the nasal cavity.

To increase oxygen flow to the cells, the right type of exercise needs to be done. This can be done by starting out slowly on a stationary bike or treadmill for no more than fifteen minutes daily. When fifteen minutes of exercise is done easily add something like stomach crunches to the routine. The goal with exercising is to retrain the muscles to accept oxygen. The key to being successful is going at a steady and consistent pace. (Shoemaker, 2010, p. 247) Over exercising will cause additional problems.

Hyperbaric Oxygen Chambers may be another way to help improve oxygen flow. There have been no studies for using the chamber this way but other studies have found positive results for other purposes. (Bhutani & Vishwanath, 2012; Pilla, Landon, & Dean, 2013)

Supplements are a good addition to any detoxification program. When I had gotten off the plane in Portland, Oregon and was sickened by the mold condition, one supplement, milk thistle, enabled me to be fully present at the conference. Milk thistle helps support the liver so that the liver is able to clear toxins. Milk thistle has antioxidant properties that protect the cells from damage caused by toxins. The dosage that worked for me was 250 mg four times a day for three days. This dosage was based on my experience and not on clinical research. The clinical trials have used a daily dose of 420 mg divided in three doses. ("Milk Thistle," 2013)

Supporting the gut helps the body's overall ability to detoxify and can help rid the body of any harmful gastrointestinal microbes. I have successfully used time released oregano oil and a multi-strain probiotic for this purpose. Oregano oil is known to be effective in the eradication of harmful microbes. The recommended oregano dose is a total of 600 mg divided into either three or four doses daily. The probiotic that I use contains Bifidobacterium breve, Bifidobacterium longum, Bifidobacterium infantis, lactobacillus acidophilus, lactobacillus plantarum, lactobacillus paracasei, lactobacillus bulgaricus and streptococcus thermophilus. There are other supplements and herbs that are helpful for someone with a mold issue.

Supplemental Suggestions

Supplement	Dosage	Reference
Berberine	200 mg two to four times daily	("Altern Med Rev," 2000; Tintu, Dileep, Tintu I, & Sadasivan, 2012)
Boswellia serrata (frankincense)	500 mg, three to four times daily	(Meletis, 2013)
Bromelain	600 mg two to four time per day on empty stomach	(Meletis, 2013)
Milk Thistle	420 mg divided into three doses	("Milk Thistle," 2013)
Ocimun sanctum (holy basil)	250 mg twice daily	(Meletis, 2013)
Oregano (time released)	600 mg divided three to four times daily	(Vasquez, 2006)
Probiotic Broad Spectrum		(Meletis, 2013)
Quercetin	2,000 mg per day	(Meletis, 2013)
Stephania tetrandra	300 mg twice daily	(Meletis, 2013)
Vitamin C	2 to 2 grams per day	(Meletis, 2013)
Vitamin D	Test for optimal levels	(Meletis, 2013)
Zingiber Officinale (ginger)	200 mg, twice daily	(Meletis, 2013)

Suggested Dietary Additions

Food/Herb/Spice	Reference
Basil	(Yin & Cheng, 1998)
Chinese parsley	(Yin & Cheng, 1998)
Garlic	(Kocić-Tanackov et al., 2012; Tedeschi, Maietti, Boggian, Vecchiati, & Brandolini, 2007; Yin & Cheng, 1998)
Green onions	(Kocić-Tanackov et al, 2012; Yin & Cheng, 1998)
Hot peppers	(Yin & Cheng, 1998)
Oregano	(Portillo-Ruiz, Sánchez, Ramos, Muñoz, & Nevárez-Moorillón, 2012)

(Kocić-Tanackov et al., 2012; Tedeschi, Maietti, Boggian, Vecchiati, & Brandolini, 2007; Yin & Cheng, 1998)

Optional steps that are not part of the conventional medical community but are believed to be helpful include some form of mind, body and spirit practice. This can be implemented with things like healthRhythms, massage and yoga to help reduce the stress caused by the illness. (http://healthrhythms.org/)

Health Coaches should be utilized to give the person someone to talk to that will listen. Many people with mold illness have been from doctor to doctor without ever having their issues addressed. Having someone who will listen will give the person enormous support throughout the healing process.

The key with any approach to curing mold illness is for the body to heal enough so that when a person unknowingly enters a contaminated building the immune response will not be so severe that the person becomes debilitated. With the right technique mold sensitive people can have their lives restored so they can live fully.

(Foster, Kane, & Speight, 2002; Shoemaker & House, 2005)

12 FICTITOUS MOLD SENSITIVITY CASE

Kim was born in the South American country of Uruguay which has a humid subtropical climate. At an early age she developed upper respiratory symptoms. After many bouts of respiratory illness, Kim had her tonsils removed. Even without her tonsils she still had symptoms.

When she was eight, her family moved to the United States. They lived in a small apartment and Kim adjusted very easily. For the first time since birth there were no respiratory issues. Kim had extremely long arms making her an excellent basketball player. She was recruited to a top college to play basketball.

Things were really going well for Kim; she graduated college amongst the top of her class with an education degree. Happily she accepted a teaching post at a local school. Within a few days after starting her teaching job, Kim started to get ill with the same respiratory illnesses that she left behind in South America so many years ago. Kim was totally caught by surprise. As this was her first job she struggled during the week to get to school. Her time on the weekend was spent recuperating. She did not have time to do the things that she liked to do. She noticed that her symptoms lessened any time she was not at work. During school holidays she even felt well enough to do some of the fun things that she now missed in her life. She went from doctor to doctor without much success. She was treated for sinus infections and given medication but none of them worked.

The other thing she noticed was that many of the students and faculty at the school had respiratory issues. One day while at school she sent a student to the custodian's office to pick up some cleaning supplies. When the student came back he reported to her that it smelled really bad in the office and there were water leaks everywhere. The custodian's office door had always been closed and usually no one saw what was going on in there. Kim immediately reported what the student found to the principal who did not seem interested in hearing about the problem.

Kim wondered if the issue in the custodian's office was related to her illness and that of others. She became friends with the custodian and learned that there was a huge mold problem in the office from leaky pipes. He had tried to get the administration to fix the problem for years but never got anywhere. One of the vents in Kim's classroom came from the custodian's office. Kim knew in her heart that what was going on in that office contributed to her illness. Armed with new information and hope she made a doctor's appointment. She was so excited to tell the doctor about the findings that she was not prepared for the response. The doctor told her that people do not get sick from mold.

All hopes of getting well again were crushed. In her heart she knew the mold was the cause but no one would listen. Back at the school she tried to get the principal to address the problem. She talked with other teachers about how their illness could be related to the condition in the custodial room. To her surprise she was reprimanded and told never to discuss this again. Kim became disheartened and asked to be transferred to another school. That request was denied.

Each day her illness escalated and most of her time during holidays was used to recover. In the two years that she was working at the school she had gained a lot of weight. Dieting and exercising did not help. Walking up stairs became a laborious task. She was constantly thirsty. Recently, she noticed that she was getting a lot of unexplained nose bleeds. A couple of times a week she would get lost while driving home. She missed playing basketball but in her state she could barely lift a ball and her muscles hurt.

Since Kim was a teacher she had summers off. This gave her body time to recuperate. Once she felt better she would go out and do the things that she missed in her life. The summer after her third year of teaching she met John. John changed her life forever. Throughout the summer they dated. It was sometimes difficult to hold hands; Kim was full of electricity often giving John a shock. They laughed about it whenever it happened. The summer ended and Kim went back to work. Like other years her health quickly deteriorated. John was shocked about the change and figured it had to do with stress from her job. One day he paid a surprise visit to Kim's school and upon entering the building he knew immediately that there was a mold problem in the school. John had an uncle with similar problems and put Kim in touch with his uncle. The uncle told her she would need to stop working at the school if she had any hopes of getting well. John's uncle also put her in touch with a doctor who specialized in mold disease. After much persistence Kim was able to transfer to a new school which was in a mold-free building. The doctor John's uncle recommended, listened to her complaints and was able to help her. Kim learned the hard way about mold disease but she was able to start the recovery process.

Although Kim is a fictional character the ending could have been quite different. Kim could have become falsely diagnosed with many wrong conditions and her health would have quickly spiraled in a negative manner until she was no longer able to work and went on disability. If the diagnosis was psychological under the current laws she would only be given two years of disability. If in the two year period of disability Kim could not find enough help for her condition so that she could return to work, there is a strong possibilty that she would lose benefits and have no source of income.

In the story Kim was reprimanded for trying to get the mold condition remedied. Unfortunately in many job situations the management does not want to address the problem. I personally experienced a similar situation with one of the companies I worked at during my career. The management chose to ignore the problem. The company eventually was forced out of embarrassment to fix the problem after an article about the situation appeared in the newspaper.

13 SUMMARY

Mold sensitivity syndrome is a complex problem. With the right diagnosis and treatment it is possible for people with mold sensitivity disease to enjoy life again. The ideal approach for handling someone with mold disease is removal from the environment that was making them ill. This will enable their body to heal without constantly getting assaulted by additional mold exposure. If the mold is not remediated, the person may experience some relief through other treatments but will be unable to detoxify properly. Ideally, a mold expert should be hired to ensure the building is cleaned correctly. Cholestyramine or butyrate can help the body detoxify and can be started while the mold problem is being remediated.

Additionally biofilm needs to be addressed. Since biofilm mostly accumulates in the nose, a nasal spray like BEG or colloidal silver is necessary to break it down.

By doing these steps the biomarkers will be controlled and the person will have less of an immunological response from accidental exposure. It is not until the biomarkers are under control that a person is able to re-enter a building that has had water damage.

Diet plays an important role in this condition as well as many others. To help control the inflammatory response associated with mold sensitivity, a gluten-free diet should be observed during the healing process. Foods that cause sensitivity should also be avoided.

Unfortunately, the time lost while victim to the disease cannot be regained. But building up the body's defenses will prevent the person from becoming chronically ill again.

No one will know until many years have passed if there are any new complications with this disease or if by adaption the next generation of people with the mold sensitive gene will be able to coexist with the mold biotoxins.

It is my hope that by reading this book you walk away with some tools to help you on your journey to recovery. One day not in the too distant future you will walk into a building and feel no discomfort to slight discomfort instead of the feeling that your health is slipping away from you. From my own personal experience after September 11th, I know this is possible and I am excited that you will soon be well enough to enjoy the things that you missed while ill.

GLOSSARY

This is a summary of some of the key terms in the book that are referenced.

Actin - A protein that is found in the muscle. When it combines with myosin it causes the muscle to contract.

Adenosine triphosphate (ATP) - Main source of energy in the cells.

Adrenal glands - Endocrine organs located on top of the kidneys, mainly responsible for releasing hormones in response to stress.

Adrenaline - Also known as epinephrine, is a hormone released from the adrenal glands during stress as part of the "Fight or Flight" mechanism.

Adrenocorticotropic hormone (ACTH) - Also known as corticotropin, is a hormone produced by the pituitary gland in response to stress.

Allergy - Hypersensitive response of the immune system to a physical or chemical agent.

Alpha melanocyte stimulating hormone (MSH) - Group of peptide hormones produced by the skin, pituitary gland and hypothalamus in response to ultraviolet radiation. It plays an important role in skin pigmentation.

Antecedents - Predisposing factors to acute and chronic illness.

Antibacterial - Anything that destroys or suppresses bacteria's growth ability.

Antibody - Protein produced by the immune system to identify and neutralize foreign objects.

Anti-diuretic hormone (ADH) - Also known as vasopressin. Hormone made by the hypothalamus (part of the brain) that helps control blood pressure and conserve fluid volume of water in the body.

Antifungal - Anything that destroys or suppresses fungus ability to grow.

Anti-gliadin antibodies - Antibody produced in response to gliadin which is an amino acid found in wheat.

Antimicrobial - Anything that destroys or suppresses a microbe's ability to grow.

Anti-neutrophil cytoplasmic antibody (ANCA) - Protein produced by the immune system. When found in blood tests it is often an indication of autoimmune disease.

Antispasmodic - Drug or herb that suppresses muscle spasms.

Apoptosis - Preprogrammed process of cell death.

Assimilation - The process of bringing required molecules from the outside into the body and incorporating them into the body's tissues.

Asthma - Common chronic inflammatory disease of the airways that makes breathing difficult.

Autoimmune disease - Abnormal immune response causing the immune system to attack healthy cells.

Bacteria - Prokaryotic microorganisms that are very small.

Bactroban - Pharmaceutical antibacterial substance.

Benlate - Also known as benomyl is a fungicide by DuPont.

Bile - Watery greenish fluid produced by the liver and stored in the gallbladder that aids in digestion of lipids.

Biofilm - Group of microorganisms joined together to form a matrix.

Biotoxin - Toxic substance produced by a living organism.

Biotransformation - Chemical modification of a compound by an organism

Blood brain barrier - Protective barrier of the brain that allows entry of beneficial substances but blocks neurotoxins.

Brassicas (Cruciferae) - Family of plants that includes cruciferous vegetables such as cabbages, broccoli and cauliflower.

Butyrate - Conjugate base of butyric acid which is a byproduct of anaerobic fermentation.

Capillaries - Small blood vessels where the actual exchange of chemicals between the blood stream and the cells occurs.

Carcinogenic - Any substance or agent that tends to produce cancer.

Cardiolipins - Common membrane protein in the body.

Caudate nucleus - Brain part that is essential for memory and learning.

Cellulose - String of sugar molecules making plant cell walls.

Cholestyramine - Cholesterol binding drug that can attach to the toxins from bile, preventing reabsorption.

Cholesterol - Fat soluble substance used by the body to form hormones. It is so important to the body that the body manufactures it. It can also be produced from food.

Circadian rhythm - The daily cycle of biological activity based on a 24 hour period. It is influenced by the environment.

Colloidal silver - Mineral that has been used to treat infections that are caused by yeast and bacteria.

Complement c4-a (C4-a) - Protein that is encoded in the C4A gene. Deficiency in this protein is associated with systemic lupus erythematosus and Type I Diabetes.

Complement system - Defense system made of many proteins that destroy microbes by causing inflammation, phagocytosis and cytolysis. These proteins also prevent cell damage.

Cortisol - Glucocorticoid steroid hormone that is produced in the adrenal cortex when the blood glucose is low and during periods of high stress.

Creosote - Gummy, combustible byproduct of wood burning that is formed when the volatile gases from the burning process combine and condense on the way out of the chimney.

Crinnion, Walter, ND - Dr. Crinnion is a pioneer in the field of Naturopathic Environmental Medicine. He specializes in treating chronic diseases that are caused by environmental toxins. He also is a bestselling author of the book "CLEAN, GREEN & LEAN: Get Rid of the Toxins That Make You Fat".

Cushing syndrome - Condition caused by hyper-secretion of glucocorticoids.

Cyanide - Lethal poison that is toxic to the mitochondria.

Cyclic adenosine monophosphate (cAMP) - Molecule formed in ATP that acts as second messenger for regulation of glycogen, sugar and lipid metabolism.

Cytokines - Small glycoproteins that are released by cell in the immune system to help regulate the immune response.

Diabetes - Condition where body can't utilize glucose correctly.

DNA - Abbreviation for deoxyribonucleic acid; is the molecule that contains the genetic code of the organism.

EDTA - Abbreviation for Ethylenediaminetetraacetic acid; is a preservative found in many foods to prevent them from spoiling too quickly.

Elimination diet - Diet designed to identify foods that may be causing an allergy or other symptoms. The diet involves removal of food from the diet for around 14 days to see if the symptoms disappear, then adding it back to see if the symptoms reappear.

Endocrine disruptor - Chemicals that interfere with the endocrine system by mimicking or blocking the action of a natural hormone.

Endorphin - Endocrine system proteins that reduce pain sensation.

Endothelial growth factor (VEGF) - Signal protein that brings homeostasis to the tissues when the oxygen supply is low from inadequate blood circulation.

Environmental Protection Agency (EPA) - Independent Federal Government agency that sets and enforces standards that protect the environment and control pollution.

Environmental relative moldiness index (ERMI) - Tool developed by the EPA to determine the potential health risks of indoor mold.

Environmental working group - Non-profit, non-partisan organization dedicated to protecting human health and the environment. They produce consumer guides like the "Dirty dozen" and the "Clean Fifteen" to help people know which foods are sprayed the most with pesticides.

Enzyme - Proteins that accelerate chemical reactions.

Fatty acid - Long-chain hydrocarbon containing a carboxyl group at one end, they are the building blocks of fat in our bodies.

Fiber - Parts of the fruits and vegetables that cannot be digested. It helps move food through the digestive tract.

Formaldehyde - A colorless foul smelling gas that is toxic and carcinogenic.

Functional medicine - A practice of medicine that is not disease based but patient centered; the underlying causes of the disease are addressed through a partnership with both the patient and the practitioner.

Fungus - Organism that feeds on organic matter.

Gamma-glutamyl transpeptidase (GGTP) - Important enzyme for bile flow that is found in many tissues especially the liver.

Gene - Biological unit of heredity that corresponds to a segment of DNA which is located on a particular chromosome.

Genotype - Genetic characteristics of an organism.

Gentamicin - Antibiotic that fights bacteria in the body.

Gliadin - Protein that is present in wheat and other cereals. It is a component of gluten.

Glucagon - Hormone produced in the pancreas that increases blood glucose levels.

Gluten - Protein in wheat and grains that is composed of gliadin and glutenin.

Gray matter - Neural tissue found in the brain and spinal cord that has a brownish gray color. It is associated with intellect.

healthRhythms - Research based group empowered drumming protocol, developed by Dr. Barry Bittman which has biological and psychosocial benefits and is a tool for communication and personal expression.

Heating, ventilation and air conditioning (HVAC) - Technology to control the indoor comfort of a building.

High-efficiency particulate absorption (HEPA) - Type of air filter that must remove 99.97% of the particles that have a size of 0.3 μm or larger.

Histone - Proteins associated with DNA in most eukaryotic organisms.

Homeostasis - Internal equilibrium maintained by the body.

Hormone - Chemical that when secreted alters the metabolic activity of target cells.

Human leukocyte antigen (HLA) – Proteins that are encoded on genes and found on cell surfaces. Plays an important role in the body's immune response to foreign invaders.

Hypothalamus - Part of the brain responsible for hormone production.

Immune system - System that protects organisms from disease.

Infection - Invasion of undesired microorganisms into the body

Inflammation - Protective mechanism in response to tissue injury designed to wall off the area.

Infrared - Invisible radiant energy that has wavelengths between 800 nanometers and 1 millimeter.

Insulin - Hormone produced in the pancreas that decreases blood glucose levels.

Intracellular signal transduction - Process where a signal is passed through a series of steps within the cell and the last step causes a change in function of the cell.

Leaky gut - Damage to the intestinal lining that allows incompletely digested proteins, fats and waste to leak out of the intestines and into the blood stream.

Leprosy - Long term contagious infection caused by bacillus Mycobacterium leprae bacteria that has been known since Biblical times.

Leptin - Hormone produced in fat tissue, signals body to stop eating.

Lyme disease - Disease caused by Borrelia burgdorferi bacteria that is attributed to tick bites from infected ticks.

Magnetic resonance imaging (MRI) - Medical imaging technique used to determine the health of the anatomy and physiology inside of the body.

MARCoNS - Abbreviation for antibiotic resistant coagulase negative staphylococci.

Matrix metallopeptidase 9 (MMP-9) - Enzyme encoded by MMP9 gene.

Mediators - Intermediaries that contribute to the presence of disease.

Melatonin - Hormone secreted by pineal gland that helps set the timing of the body's biological clock.

Microbial volatile organic compounds (MVOC) - Microbes that produce volatile organic compounds.

Microorganisms - Organism of microscopic size.

Minimum efficiency reporting value (MERV) - Rating for the effectiveness of air filters.

Mitochondria - Part of the cell responsible for oxidizing glucose to produce energy for the cell use.

Mold - Growth produced by fungus on damp or decaying organic matter or living organisms.

Mold sensitivity syndrome - An acute and chronic health condition that occurs after being exposed to mold usually from a water damaged building.

Mold specific quantitative PCR (MSQPCR) - Comparison to a national database of the mold in a building.

Mucous membranes - Membranes that line the body cavities that opens to the exterior.

Mycotoxin - Secondary metabolites produced by a fungus, capable of causing disease.

Neti Pot - Container designed to clean the nasal cavity.

Neuroendocrinology - Study of the interactions between the endocrine system and the nervous system.

Neuroquant® - Computer program used for people with traumatic brain injury to measure brain volume.

Neurotoxin - Substance that inhibits nervous system cell function.

No-amylose diet - Diet that eliminates foods that contain high concentrations of amylose. Amylose is a polysaccharide similar to glucose.

Origanum syriacum - Herb in the mint family.

Ozonated water - Cold water that is infused with ozone to purify it.

Pathogen - Disease producing microbe.

Plague - An infectious disease that infects many people that is caused by bacteria and often causes death to large groups of people.

Plasminogen activator inhibitor-1 (PAI-1) - Protein that is encoded by the SERPINE1 gene that regulates the fibrinolytic system. The fibrinolytic system is responsible for breaking down blood clots.

Plasticizers - Substances that when added to a chemical, make it more flexible, workable or stretchable.

Polychlorinated biphenyl (PCB) – Toxic man-made chlorinated hydrocarbons, banned for commercial production in the United States.

Prednisone - Glucocorticoid Pharmaceutical drug that is commonly used for its anti-inflammatory activity.

Protein kinase - An enzyme that modifies other cellular proteins.

Proteolysis - Breaking down of proteins.

PubMed - Free online resource for searching biomedical literature.

Retina - Light sensitive layer of tissue that lines the surface of the eye.

Scarlet - In Biblical times it was red dyed wool.

September 11, 2001 - Day terrorists attacked New York City and Washington, DC causing the loss of lives, destruction of the World Trade Center Towers, 7 World Trade Center, Pentagon damage and a downed plane in Pennsylvania.

Shoemaker, Ritchie, MD – Biotoxin related illness pioneer in research, patient care and education.

Sick Building Syndrome (SBS) - Building occupants become ill while spending time in the building but feel better upon leaving.

Steroid - Type of organic compound that is in the body, notably as hormones and cholesterol. It is also used in many pharmaceutical drugs.

Steroidogenesis - The process that creates steroids.

Tea tree oil - Oil obtained from the leaves of the Melaleuca tree. It is topical antimicrobial.

Thieves essential oil - Essential oil from a mixture of cinnamon, clove, eucalyptus, lemon and rosemary. It is known for its cleansing properties and support of the immune system.

Transforming growth factor (TGF) - Also known as tumor growth factor are the proteins that stimulate the normal cell growth.

Triggers - Events or entities that provoke the disease or its symptoms.

Ultraviolet - Type of radiation with a wave length between visible light and x-rays.

Vasoactive intestinal polypeptide (VIP) - Hormone that regulates cytokine response, pulmonary artery pressure and inflammatory response.

Vasopressin – see Anti-diuretic hormone (ADH)

Visual contrast sensitivity (VCS) - Screening test to determine the possibilty of toxins based on neurologic functions of vision known as contrast.

Vo2 max - Maximum rate of oxygen consumption measured during exercise.

Volatile organic compounds (VOC) - Chemicals that have a low molecular weight, low water solubility and high vapor pressure and therefore can evaporate easily into the air or "off-gas".

White blood cells - Cells of the immune system that protect the body from disease and foreign invaders.

White matter - Myelinated nerve fibers that regulate electrical signals in axons. Myelin is an insulator gives the white matter its white color.

World health organization (WHO) - Specialized agency of the United Nations that is concerned with International public health.

REFERENCES

Akpinar-Elci, M., White, S. K., Siegel, P. D., Park, J. H., Visotcky, A., Kreiss, K., & Cox-Ganser, J. M. (2013, February 6). Markers of upper airway inflammation associated with microbial exposure and symptoms in occupants of a water-damaged building. *American Journal of Industrial Medicine*. Retrieved from http://www.ncbi.nlm.nih.gov/pubmed/23390064

Attfield, M. D., Cox-Ganser, J. M., Kreiss, K., & Park, J. (2004, December). Building-related respiratory symptoms can be predicted with semi-quantitative indices of exposure to dampness and mold. *Indoor Air*, *14*(6), 425-433. Retrieved from http://www.ncbi.nlm.nih.gov/pubmed/15500636

Bakkour, Y., Kasir, S., Kanj, D., Omar, F. E., & Mouneimne, Y. (2011). Analysis of the essential oils of Salvia Libanotica Analysis of the essential oils of Salvia Libanotica and Origanum Syriacum. *Journal of Natural Products*, 4, 51-56. Retrieved from http://journalofnaturalproducts.com/Volume4/8_Res_paper-7.pdf

Barmark, M. (2014, Nov 26). Social determinants of the sick building syndrome: exploring the interrelated effects of social position and psychosocial situation. *International Journal of Environmental Health Research*, 1-18.

Berberine. (2000, April). *Altern Med Rev*, *5*(2), 175-7. Retrieved from http://www.thorne.com/altmedrev/.fulltext/5/2/175.pdf

Bhutani, S., & Vishwanath, G. (2012, May). Hyperbaric oxygen and wound healing. *Indian J Plast Surg, 45*(2), 316-324. Retrieved from http://www.ncbi.nlm.nih.gov/pubmed/23162231

Brennan, A. M., & Mantzoros, C. S. (2006, June). Drug Insight: the role of leptin in human physiology and pathophysiology--emerging clinical applications. *Nature Clinical Practice Endocrinology & Metabolism,* 2(6), 318–327. http://dx.doi.org/10.1038/ncpendmet0196

Cheong, C. (2014, Feb). A proper strategy for combating mould. *Health Estate, 68*(2), 17-20.

Cháfer, M., Sánchez-González, L., González-Martínez, C., & Chiralt, A. (2012, August). Fungal decay and shelf life of oranges coated with chitosan and bergamot, thyme, and tea tree essential oils. *Journal Food Science, 77*(8), 182-187. Retrieved from http://www.ncbi.nlm.nih.gov/pubmed/22860582

Crinnion, W. (2010). *Clean, Green, and Lean.* Hoboken, NJ: John Wiley & Sons, Inc.

Crinnion, W. J. (2012, March). Do environmental toxicants contribute to allergy and asthma? *Alternative Medicine Review, 17*(1), 6-18. Retrieved from http://www.altmedrev.com/publications/17/1/6.pdf

Ebbehøj, N. E., Meyer, H. W., Würtz, H., Suadicani, P., Valbjørn, O., Sigsgaard, T., & Gyntelberg, F. (2005). Molds in floor dust, building-related symptoms, and lung function among male and female schoolteachers. *Indoor Air, 15*(Suppl 10), 7-16. Retrieved from http://www.ncbi.nlm.nih.gov/pubmed/15926939

Esposito, S., Prada, E., Mastrolla, M. V., Tarantino, G., Codeca, C., & Rigante, D. (2014, Nov 14). Autoimmune/inflammatory syndrome induced by adjuvants (ASIA): clues and pitfalls in the pediatric background. *Immunologic Research.* http://dx.doi.org/10.1007/s12026-014-8586-0

Forrer, M., Kulik, E. M., Filippi, A., & Waltimo, T. (2013, January). The antimicrobial activity of alpha-bisabolol and tea tree oil against Solobacterium moorei, a Gram-positive bacterium associated with halitosis. *Archives of Oral Biology, 58*(1), 10-16. http://dx.doi.org/10.1016/j.archoralbio.2012.08.001

Foster, J., Kane, P., & Speight, N. (2002, November). The Detoxx™ System: Detoxification of Biotoxins in Chronic Neurotoxic Syndromes. *Townsend Letter for Doctors & Patients*. Retrieved from http://www.townsendletter.com/Nov_2002/detoxxsystem1102.htm

Friedman, J. M., & Halaas, J. L. (1998). Leptin and the regulation of body weight in mammals. *Nature, 395*(6704), 763–770. http://dx.doi.org/10.1038/27376

Frizzell, C., Verhaegen, S., Ropstad, E., Elliott, C. T., & Connolly, L. (2013, March 13). Endocrine disrupting effects of ochratoxin A at the level of nuclear receptor activation and steroidogenesis. *Toxicology Letters, 217*(3), 243-50. http://dx.doi.org/10.1016/j.toxlet.2012.12.018

Fung, F., & Hughson, W. (2008, April). The Fundamentals of Mold-Related Illness -When to suspect the environment is making a patient sick. *Cardiovascular Events, 120*(1).

Fusunyan, R. D., Quinn, J. J., Ohno, Y., MacDermott, R. P., & Sanderson, I. R. (1998, January). Butyrate enhances interleukin (IL)-8 secretion by intestinal epithelial cells in response to IL-1beta and lipopolysaccharide. *Pediatric Research, 43*(1), 84-90. Retrieved from http://www.ncbi.nlm.nih.gov/pubmed/9432117

GUNNBJÖRNSDOTTIR, M. I., NORBÄCK, D., PLASCHKE, P., NORRMAN, E., BJÖRNSSON, E., & JANSON, C. (2003, May). The relationship between indicators of building dampness and respiratory health in young Swedish adults. *Respiratory Medicine*,

97(4), 302-307. Retrieved from
http://www.ncbi.nlm.nih.gov/pubmed/11401019

Gray, M. (2006, April 19-22). *Molds and Mycotoxins: Beyond Allergies and Asthma...* Paper presented at the 13th International Symposium of The Institute for Functional Medicine, Tampa, FL. Abstract retrieved from http://www.alternative-therapies.com/at/web_pdfs/ifm_proceedings_low.pdf

Hudnell, K., House, D. E., & Shoemaker, R. (2003, September 10 - December 03). *VISUAL CONTRAST SENSITIVITY: A SENSITIVE INDICATOR OF NEUROTOXICITY FOR RISK ASSESSMENT AND CLINICAL APPLICATIONS.* . Paper presented at the 5th International Conference on Bioaerosols, Fungi, Bacteria, Mycotoxins and Human Health, Saratoga Spring, NY. Abstract retrieved from http://cfpub.epa.gov/si/si_public_record_Report.cfm?dirEntryId =76427&CFID=109246433&CFTOKEN=68463011&jsessionid= 383092a375a9b6d57f805820252245765866

Jones, D. S., & Quinn, S. (Eds.). (2010). *Textbook of Functional Medicine.* Gig Harbor, WA: The Institute of Functional Medicine.

Karunasena, E., Larrañaga, M. D., Simoni, J. S., Douglas, D. R., & Straus, D. C. (2010, December). Building-associated neurological damage modeled in human cells: a mechanism of neurotoxic effects by exposure to mycotoxins in the indoor environment. *Mycopathologia, 170*(6), 377-390. http://dx.doi.org/10.1007/s11046-010-9330-5

Kim, J. L., Elfman, L., Mi, Y., Wieslander, G., Smedje, G., & Norback, D. (2007, April). Indoor molds, bacteria, microbial volatile organic compounds and plasticizers in schools – associations with asthma and respiratory symptoms in pupils. *Indoor Air, 17*(2), 153-163. http://dx.doi.org/10.1111/j.1600-0668.2006.00466.x

Kocić-Tanackov, S., Dime, G., Lević, J., Tanackov, I., Tepić, A., Vujičić, B., & Gvozdanović-Varga, J. (2012, May). Effects of onion (Allium cepa L.) and garlic (Allium sativum L.) essential oils on the Aspergillus versicolor growth and sterigmatocystin production. *J Food Sci.*, *77*(5), M278-84. http://dx.doi.org/0.1111/j.1750-3841.2012.02662.x

Kustrzeba-Wojcicka, I., Siwak, E., Terlecki, G., Wolanczyk-Medrala, A., & Medrala, W. (2014, September 10). Alternaria alternata and Its Allergens: a Comprehensive Review. *Clinical Review in Allergy and Immunology*, *47*, 354-365. http://dx.doi.org/10.1007/s12016-014-8447-6

Li, C. S., Hsu, C. W., & Lu, C. H. (1997, Jan-Feb). Dampness and respiratory symptoms among workers in daycare centers in a subtropical climate. *Archives of Environmental Health*, *52*(1), 68-71. Retrieved from http://www.ncbi.nlm.nih.gov/pubmed/9039861

Lin, Z. M., Zhao, J. X., Duan, X. N., Zhang, L. B., Ye, J. M., Xu, L., & Liu, Y. H. (2014). Effects of tissue factor, PAR-2 and MMP-9 expression on human breast cancer cell line MCF-7 invasion. *Asian Pacific Journal of Cancer Prevention*, *15*(2), 643-646. http://dx.doi.org/10.7314/APJCP.2014.15.2.643

Margetic, S., Gazzola, C., Pegg, G. G., & Hill, R. A. (2002). Leptin: a review of its peripheral actions and interactions. *International Journal of Obesity and Related Metabolic Disorders*, *26*(11), 1407–1433.

Meklin, T., Husman, T., Vepsalainen, A., Vahteristo, M., Koivisto, J., Halla-Aho, J., Nevalainen, A. (2002, September). Indoor air microbes and respiratory symptoms of children in moisture damaged and reference schools. *Indoor Air*, *12*(3), 175-183. Retrieved from http://www.ncbi.nlm.nih.gov/pubmed/12244747

Meklin, T., Hyvärinen, A., Toivola, M., Reponen, T., Koponen, V., Husman, T., ... Nevalainen, A. (2003, Jan-Feb). Effect of building frame and moisture damage on microbiological indoor air quality in school buildings. *AIHA J*, *64*(1), 108-116. Retrieved from http://www.ncbi.nlm.nih.gov/pubmed/12570403

Meklin, T., Potus, T., Pekkanen, J., Hyvärinen, A., Hirvonen, M. R., & Nevalainen, A. (2005). Effects of moisture-damage repairs on microbial exposure and symptoms in schoolchildren. *Indoor Air*, *15*(Suppl 10), 40-47. Retrieved from http://www.ncbi.nlm.nih.gov/pubmed/15926943

Meletis, C. (2013, March). Black Mold: The Great Pretender. *Complementary Prescriptions Journal*, *27*(3), 1, 7-8.

Milk Thistle. (2013). *American Botanical Council.*

Mold. (2013). In *the Merriam-Webster Unabridged Dictionary*. Retrieved from http://www.merriam-webster.com/dictionary/mold

Monteiro, D. R., Silva, S., Negri, M., Gorup, L. F., De Camargo, E. R., Oliveira, R., ... Henriques, M. (2012, Dec 12). Silver colloidal nanoparticles: effect on matrix composition and structure of Candida albicans and Candida glabrata biofilms. *J Appl Microbiol.* http://dx.doi.org/10.1111/jam.12102

Nielsen, K. F. (2003, March 6). Mycotoxin production by indoor molds. *Fungal Genetics and Biology*, *39*, 103–117. Retrieved from http://www.nchh.org/Portals/0/Contents/Article0231.pdf

Park, J., Cox-Ganser, J. M., Kreiss, K., White, S. K., & Rao, C. Y. (2007, January). Hydrophilic Fungi and Ergosterol Associated with Respiratory Illness in a Water-Damaged Building. *Environmental Health Perspectives*, *116*(1), 45-50. Retrieved from http://www.ncbi.nlm.nih.gov/pubmed/18197298

Pilla, R., Landon, C. S., & Dean, J. B. (2013, Feb 21). A potential early physiological marker for CNS oxygen toxicity: hyperoxic hyperpnea precedes seizure in unanesthetized rats breathing hyperbaric oxygen. *J Appl Physiol.* Retrieved from http://www.ncbi.nlm.nih.gov/pubmed/23429869

Portillo-Ruiz, M. C., Sánchez, R. A., Ramos, S. V., Muñoz, J. V., & Nevárez-Moorillón, G. V. (2012, August). Antifungal effect of Mexican oregano (Lippia berlandieri Schauer) essential oil on a wheat flour-based medium. *J Food Sci.*, *77*(8), M441-5. http://dx.doi.org/10.1111/j.1750-3841.2012.02821.x

Rao, C. Y., Cox-Ganser, J. M., Chew, G. L., Doekes, G., & White, S. (2005, May). Use of surrogate markers of biological agents in air and settled dust samples to evaluate a water-damaged hospital. *Indoor Air*, *15*(s9), 89-97. Retrieved from http://www.ncbi.nlm.nih.gov/pubmed/15910534

Sahlberg, B., Gunnbjörnsdottir, M., Soon, A., Jogi, R., Gislason, T., Wieslander, G., Norback, D. (2013, February). Airborne molds and bacteria, microbial volatile organic compounds (MVOC), plasticizers and formaldehyde in dwellings in three North European cities in relation to sick building syndrome (SBS). *Science of the Total Environment*, *444*(1), 433-440. Retrieved from http://www.sciencedirect.com/science/article/pii/S0048969712014775

Santo-Pietro, K. A. (206, April). Microbial Volatile Organic Compounds (MVOC's). *The Environmental Reporter*, *4*(4). Retrieved from https://www.emlab.com/s/sampling/env-report-04-2006.html

Savilahti, R., Uitti, J., Laippala, P., Husman, T., & Roto, P. (2000, Nov-Dec). Respiratory Morbidity among Children Following Renovation of a Water-Damaged School. *Archives of Environmental Health*, *55*(6), 405--410. Retrieved from http://www.ncbi.nlm.nih.gov/pubmed/11128878

Savilahti, R., Uitti, J., Roto, P., Laippala, P., & Husman, T. (2001, February). Increased prevalence of atopy among children exposed to mold in a school building. *Allergy*, *56*(2), 175--179. Retrieved from http://www.ncbi.nlm.nih.gov/pubmed/11167380

Scheel, C. M., Rosing, W. C., & Farone, A. L. (2001, Sep-Oct). Possible sources of sick building syndrome in a Tennessee middle school. *Arch Environ Health, 56*(5), 413-417. Retrieved from http://www.ncbi.nlm.nih.gov/pubmed/11777022

Seuri, M., Husman, K., Kinnunen, H., Reiman, M., Kreus, R., Kuronen, P., ... Paananen, M. (2000, September). An outbreak of respiratory diseases among workers at a water-damaged building--a case report. *Indoor Air, 10*(3), 138-145. Retrieved from http://www.ncbi.nlm.nih.gov/pubmed/10979195

Shoemaker, MD, R. (2009). Episode 235 - Ritchie Shoemaker, M. D. [*IAQ Radio*. Retrieved from http://www.iaqradio.com/blog.htm

Shoemaker, R. (2010). *Surviving Mold*. Baltimore, MD: Otter Bay Books, LLC.

Shoemaker, R. (2010-2013). NeuroQuant Links Mold Illness to Structural Change in Brain. Retrieved March 2, 2013, from http://www.survivingmold.com/news/2012/10/neuroquant-links-mold-illness-to-structural-change-in-brain/

Shoemaker, R. C. (2005). *Lose the Weight You Hate*. Baltimore, MD: Gateway Press, Inc.

Shoemaker, R. C., & House, D. E. (2005, Jan-Feb). A time-series study of sick building syndrome: chronic, biotoxin-associated illness from exposure to water-damaged buildings. *Neurotoxicology Teratology, 27*(1), 29-46. Retrieved from http://www.ncbi.nlm.nih.gov/pubmed/15681119

Speight, N. (2006, September 15). BUTYRATE. *Dr Neal's House Call, 2*(25). Retrieved from http://www.cfwellness.com/articles/butyrate

Tedeschi, P., Maietti, A., Boggian, M., Vecchiati, G., & Brandolini, V. (2007, September-October). Fungitoxicity of lyophilized and spray-dried garlic extracts. *Journal of Environmental Science and Health, Part B.*,

42(7), 795-9. Retrieved from
http://www.ncbi.nlm.nih.gov/pubmed/17763036

Thomas, G., Burton, N. C., Mueller, C., Page, E., & Vesper, S. (2012, Sep).
Comparison of work-related symptoms and visual contrast
sensitivity between employees at a severely water-damaged school
and a school without significant water damage. *American Journal of
Industrial Medicine*, *55*(9), 844-854.
http://dx.doi.org/10.1002/ajim.22059

Tintu, I., Dileep, K. V., Tintu I, Dileep KV, Augustine, A., & Sadasivan, C.
(2012, October). An isoquinoline alkaloid, berberine, can inhibit
fungal alpha amylase: enzyme kinetic and molecular modeling
studies. *Chem Biol Drug Des*, *80*(4), 554-560.
http://dx.doi.org/10.1111/j.1747-0285.2012.01426.x

Tuomainen, A., Seuri, M., & Sieppi, A. (2004, April). Indoor air quality and
health problems associated with damp floor coverings. *International
Archives of Occupational and Environmental Health*, *77*(3), 222-226.
Retrieved from http://www.ncbi.nlm.nih.gov/pubmed/14689309

Vasquez, A. (2006, January). Reducing Pain and Inflammation Naturally.
Part 6: Nutritional and Botanical Treatments Against "Silent
Infections" and Gastrointestinal Dysbiosis, Commonly Overlooked
Causes of Neuromusculoskeletal Inflammation and Chronic Health
Problems. *Journal of the Council on Nutrition of the American Chiropractic
Association*.

Vesley, K. (2012, April 3). Mold Cases Prove Persistent—Will Landlords
Cough Up Cash for Little Black Spot Suits? *The New York Observer*.
Retrieved from http://observer.com/2012/04/mold-cases-prove-
persistent-will-landlords-cough-up-cash-for-little-black-spot-suits/

Wolff, H., Mussalo-Rauhamaa, H., Raitio, H., Elg, P., Orpana, A., Piilonen,
A., & Haahtela, T. (2009, September). Patients referred to an
indoor air health clinic: exposure to water-damaged buildings
causes an increase of lymphocytes in bronchoalveolar lavage and a

decrease of CD19 leucocytes in peripheral blood. *Scandinavian Journal of Clinical & Laboratory Investigation, 69*(5), 537-544. Retrieved from http://www.ncbi.nlm.nih.gov/pubmed/19347744

Wålinder, R., Norbäck, D., Wieslander, G., Smedje, G., Erwall, C., & Venge, P. (2001, March). Acoustic rhinometry and lavage biomarkers in relation to some building characteristics in Swedish schools. *Indoor Air, 11*(1). Retrieved from http://www.ncbi.nlm.nih.gov/pubmed/11235228

Yang, C., Chiu, J., Chiu, H., & Kao, W. (1997, August). Damp housing conditions and respiratory symptoms in primary school children. *Pediatric Pulmonology, 24*(2), 73-77. Retrieved from http://www.ncbi.nlm.nih.gov/pubmed/9292897

Yin, M. C., & Cheng, W. S. (1998, January). Inhibition of Aspergillus niger and Aspergillus flavus by some herbs and spices. *Journal of Food Protection, 61*(1), 123-5. Retrieved from http://www.ncbi.nlm.nih.gov/pubmed/9708267

INDEX

water · 2, 3, 4, 7, 9, 11, 12, 13, 14, 16, 17, 18, 20, 23, 24, 29, 30, 31, 33, 34, 36, 37, 38, 39, 42, 43, 46, 50, 53, 55, 62, 63, 65, 66, 71, 72, 73, 74
wet vacuums · 16
wheat · 1, 45, 56, 60, 72
white blood cells · 26, 29, 65
white matter · 28, 65
Wilhelm Mohorn · 31
wood · 6, 14, 38, 58
World Health Organization · 23, 33
World Trade Center · i, 2, 64, 91

Y

yams · 44
yoga · 48

ABOUT THE AUTHOR

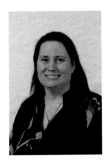

Karen Wright is a functional nutritionist, traditional naturopath and a Transformational Health Coach. She uses an integration of scientific research, biological and nutritional sciences, clinical nutrition assessment and personalized nutrition therapies to achieve optimal health, healing and vitality. Since becoming extremely ill from toxins after the Sept 11th World Trade Center attacks, Karen is very passionate about educating others about foods that support the body.

Karen is a contributing author to the book "Visionaries with Guts". She herself is a visionary who has never let obstacles get in the way of accomplishing her goals. Born dyslexic, she successfully earned a Masters of Science in Human Nutrition and Functional Medicine from the University of Western States and a doctor of traditional naturopathy from Clayton College of Natural Health.

Her education did not stop there; she obtained certification as a Health Coach from the Institute of Integrative Nutrition. Karen is certified as a Certified Master in the Transformational Coaching Method, a HealthRHYTHMS facilitator which is an evidenced based protocol using drums to create a community and enhance immune function while finding a personal inner rhythm. She is trained as a detoxification specialist and Ulan Nutritional Systems Nutrition Response Testing[SM] practitioner. She is Board Certified by the American Association of Drugless Practitioners.

Having worked in corporate America, as a research analyst, a computer programmer and manager; Karen is familiar with challenges people face daily on their jobs. She is a frequent speaker at corporate events, giving men and woman the tools to move up the corporate ladder and improve their health. Karen's career enables her to utilize her strengths while keeping her passions alive. Her actions inspire people to take chances and follow their dreams.

She lives with her two children and enjoys creating healthy meals which she shares with family members and friends.

Made in the USA
Lexington, KY
09 February 2018